# TAKING CHARGE
# OF ASTHMA

# TAKING CHARGE OF ASTHMA

## A Lifetime Strategy

Betty B. Wray, M.D.

John Wiley & Sons, Inc.

New York • Chichester • Weinheim • Brisbane • Singapore • Toronto

This text is printed on acid-free paper. ∞

Copyright © 1998 by Elizabeth A. Ryan. All rights reserved.
Published by John Wiley & Sons, Inc.
Published simultaneously in Canada.

No part of this publication may be reproduced, stored in a retrieval system or transmitted in any form or by any means, electronic, mechanical, photocopying, recording, scanning, or otherwise, except as permitted under Sections 107 or 108 of the 1976 United States Copyright Act, without either the prior written permission of the Publisher, or authorization through payment of the appropriate per-copy fee to the Copyright Clearance Center, 22 Rosewood Drive, Danvers, MA 01923, (508) 750-8400, fax (508) 750-4744. Requests to the Publisher for permission should be addressed to the Permission Department, John Wiley & Sons, Inc., 605 Third Avenue, New York, NY 10158-0012, (212) 850-6011, fax (212) 850-6008, E-Mail: PERMREQ@WILEY.COM

The information contained in this book is not intended to serve as a replacement for professional medical advice. Any use of the information in this book is at the reader's discretion. The author and publisher specifically disclaim any and all liability arising directly or indirectly from the use or application of any information contained in this book. A health care professional should be consulted regarding your specific situation.

*Library of Congress Cataloging-in-Publication Data*

Wray, Betty B.
    Taking charge of asthma : a lifetime strategy / Betty B. Wray.
       p.   cm.
    Includes index.
    ISBN 0-471-24704-9 (pbk. : alk. paper)
    1. Asthma–Popular works.   I. Title.
RC591.W73    1998
616.2'38–dc21                                                                97-48749

Printed in the United States of America

10  9  8  7  6  5  4  3  2

# Table of Contents

| | | |
|---|---|---|
| | Introduction | vii |
| 1 | How Much Do You Really Know About Asthma? | 1 |
| 2 | The Way *Your* Asthma Works: How Your Body Reacts, The Different Kinds, and Diagnosis | 15 |
| 3 | You Can Take Action | 41 |
| 4 | Understanding the Allergy-Asthma Connection | 60 |
| 5 | Coping With Your Allergies | 73 |
| 6 | Breathe Easier: Controlling Your Environment | 84 |
| 7 | Occupational Hazards and Air Pollution | 101 |
| 8 | Nourishing Your Mind, Body, and Spirit: A Holistic Approach | 109 |
| 9 | Breathing Well: Exercise Your Lungs | 125 |
| 10 | Alternative Strategies for Treating Asthma | 140 |
| 11 | Working With Your Doctor | 149 |
| 12 | Making the Most of the Least Medications | 157 |
| 13 | Children and Asthma: What Every Parent Needs to Know | 176 |

TABLE OF CONTENTS

| | | |
|---|---|---|
| Appendix A | Glossary of Terms Relating to Asthma | 199 |
| Appendix B | Food Groups | 205 |
| Appendix C | Medications and Asthma | 211 |
| Appendix D | National Organizations Dealing with Asthma and Lung-Related Disorders | 216 |
| Appendix E | National Treatment Centers (Adult and Pediatric) | 219 |
| Appendix F | Allergy Supplies | 222 |
| Appendix G | Bibliography | 223 |
| Index | | 224 |

# Introduction

Welcome to *Taking Charge of Asthma*—a comprehensive, holistic approach to managing your or your child's asthma.

As you probably know all too well by now, asthma is considered a condition that can't be cured. That is, there is no medication or treatment that permanently removes the physical basis for asthma or that permanently eliminates the possibility that a person will have an attack.

The good news, however, is that there are a great many ways that asthma can be controlled, managed, and lived with, so that the adult or child with asthma feels few or no ill effects from the condition. *Taking Charge of Asthma* will help you understand these approaches to limiting and controlling asthma, to coping with and preventing asthma attacks. This book offers a unique perspective that combines the latest in medical research with the most effective holistic techniques, incorporating diet, exercise, and lifestyle changes into an overall program for health.

There are three basic principles shaping *Taking Charge of Asthma*:

1. Your mind and your body are deeply connected.
2. Every aspect of your health affects every other aspect.
3. Knowledge is power and will help you to work with your physician to utilize treatment in the most effective way.

What this means in practice is that while medication can be a crucial part of any treatment plan, medication alone is often not enough. This book will help you work with your doctor to develop a treatment plan that probably includes some reliance on medication but that also helps you discover the diet, the exercise pattern, and the lifestyle that best support your overall health—thereby reducing the frequency and intensity of your asthma attacks. This book will likewise help you discover the attitudes

## INTRODUCTION

toward your body and your life that best support your health, so that all of you—mind, body, and emotions—can work together to prevent, reduce, control, and manage your asthma.

If your concern is a child with asthma, *Taking Charge of Asthma* will likewise help you develop an approach that takes into account all aspects of your child: teaching him or her how to use an inhaler correctly; discovering the diet that is right for him or her; dealing with family issues that might be affecting you, your spouse, and your other children; helping your child find ways to participate actively in sports, school, and social time with friends. This book will also help you figure out constructive ways to work with your physician, so that together you can come up with a treatment program that is effective for your child.

Having a chronic condition such as asthma can feel overwhelming, both to the adult or child with asthma and to the person's family. Knowing that there are short- and long-term steps you can take to manage this condition is often the first step to finding relief. Knowing that a person with asthma can indeed live a "normal," active, enjoyable life can likewise ease the pain, fear, and frustration that often accompany this persistent condition.

My research as well as my own clinical experience confirms that people with asthma can look forward to healthy, happy lives—if they understand their condition and approach it effectively. *Taking Charge of Asthma* can help you discover the approach that works best for you. I wish you well on your journey to greater health.

# 1

# How Much Do You Really Know about Asthma?

Lydia is twenty-four years old and works in a bakery. For the past several weeks, she's been coughing and wheezing at work, and it doesn't stop until just before bedtime. The problem seems to clear up on weekends and vacations, but during the workweek, she feels as though she's continually trying to catch her breath. Lydia used to go to the gym regularly after work, but since this shortness of breath started, she just doesn't feel able to exercise. Once, when she was running on the treadmill, she felt like she was suffocating, and she had to stop and cough for several minutes before she could again breathe normally. She's tried taking cough medicine, which helps for an hour or so, but then the cough comes back worse than ever—and she's started to worry about the amount of cough medicine she takes.

Lately, Lydia wakes up in the middle of the night, coughing and gasping for breath, so she's come to dread bedtime. She's also coughing and wheezing on weekends. Lydia hates to go to a doctor for such a small thing—after all, she doesn't have a fever or any other symptoms—but she's starting to feel as though this cough has completely taken over her life.

Paul is ten years old. He's had asthma ever since he can remember. Life for Paul is alternately frustrating and terrifying—either hedged about with things he can't do, or filled with hidden dangers. Paul can't visit the homes of his friends—it's too likely that he'll get an asthma attack as a result of being exposed to a pet, some household dust, a moldy basement, or a plant in the backyard. Paul can't be involved in sports—exercise makes him wheeze. He can't even relax when he goes to bed—he has too many vivid memories of waking in the middle of the night and feeling as though his pillow were being held over his face, shutting out his breath.

School is another minefield. Paul is afraid of getting an asthma attack from chalk dust, the formaldehyde in the science lab, the plants in the classroom window, or the class pet, a guinea pig who lives in a cage on the windowsill. Although Paul has an inhaler and knows how to use it to prevent asthma attacks, school rules forbid him to carry his own medication or to give it to his classroom teacher. The inhaler has to stay with the school nurse, which means that whenever Paul feels an attack coming on, he has to tell his teacher, who then has to write him a hall pass that will allow him to walk to the nurse's office. If the nurse is on break or with another student, Paul might have to wait for a while—even though he's supposed to use his inhaler right away. Just knowing that help is so far away and so uncertain makes Paul feel nervous all the time.

Malcolm, age thirty-five, has had asthma since childhood—and he's very proud that he has never let the disease interfere with his life. Malcolm has always loved basketball, which he's played ever since he was a kid and which he continues to play with a group of friends on weekends. He has vivid childhood memories of making a basket, waving to a cheering crowd, and reaching for his inhaler so that he could go right on with the game. Malcolm has a few food allergies—he reacts violently to both peanuts and shrimp—but he can easily avoid those foods. He also has intense allergic reactions to cats and dogs. Just being in a room where a pet has been can make Malcolm's throat close up and his nose start to run. A minute later, he's sneezing vigorously, coughing up mucus, and, sometimes, feeling his chest constrict. For years, Malcolm solved that problem simply by not owning a pet. And always, if an asthma attack threatened, Malcolm felt secure in the knowledge that a few puffs of his trusty inhaler would fix him right up.

Now, however, the inhaler doesn't seem to be working so well. Malcolm finds himself using it more and more often, which makes him very uneasy. His doctor has suggested adding a corticosteroid that can be inhaled. But Malcolm has read about the powerful side effects of steroids, and he's not sure that he wants to take that risk.

Meanwhile, Malcolm's wife is losing patience with him. He has always refused to enter his in-laws' house because they have two cats and a dog. Now Malcolm and his wife have a baby, and when they go to visit her parents, Malcolm waits on the porch while the others gather inside. The in-laws are sure that Malcolm's asthma is just a psychological problem—his way of avoiding family visits—and his formerly understanding wife is beginning to wonder if maybe her parents aren't right. Malcolm feels that his asthma, once so comfortably under control, is affecting his life far more than he wants it to.

Angela, age fifty-five, had always been fairly healthy, but suddenly, she's frequently ill—and when she isn't actually sick, she's exhausted, which is almost worse than being sick. All winter, she's had one infection after another: two bouts of bronchitis, a sore throat, a low-grade flu, a stuffy head cold, and constant trouble with her sinuses. Lately, Angela has been having chest pains, and when she goes out into the cold winter air, she sometimes has trouble breathing. When she complains to her doctor, his response is "Oh, everyone slows down when they get older." But Angela knows lots of people in their sixties and seventies who seem to have more energy than she does. Is she really doomed to a life of constant illness and exhaustion?

# The Many Faces of Asthma

Lydia, Paul, Malcolm, and Angela all suffer from asthma, a chronic lung disease that takes a wide variety of forms. Lydia suffers from *occupational asthma,* caused by sensitivity to wheat flour that she inhales. Paul has *childhood asthma,* the disease that begins in childhood. Malcolm's asthma began in childhood and has been relatively inactive at times, but he is becoming more highly allergic. And Angela has *adult-onset asthma,* a form of the disease that first appears in adulthood, often as late as age fifty, sixty, or even later, and is frequently accompanied by chronic sinusitis.

Asthma is one of the most common chronic diseases in the United States—and one of the most misunderstood. Let's start by sorting through some of the most prevalent myths about asthma. Take the following quiz to test your knowledge of this familiar but poorly understood disease. Then read on to separate the myths from the truths.

### *Asthma Myths and Truths*

Underline, circle, or check your responses to these questions:

1. Asthma is primarily psychological in origin. When a person has eliminated the stress in his or her life, asthma tends to disappear.

   True        False

2. Most children who have asthma outgrow the disease by adulthood.

   True        False

3. There are two basic types of asthma: *intrinsic,* caused by internal biological factors, and *extrinsic,* caused by reactions to allergens and environmental factors.

   True        False

4. You are at increased risk of getting asthma if someone in your family has it.

   True        False

# How Much Do You Really Know about Asthma?

5. You are far more likely to develop asthma if you live with someone (e.g., a spouse or a roommate) who has the disease.

    True                False

6. Which, if any, of the following factors is likely to cause people to develop asthma?

    a. smoking
    b. overeating
    c. lack of exercise
    d. too much exercise
    e. stress

7. Which, if any, of the following factors is likely to trigger an asthma attack in a person who has already had at least one asthma attack?

    a. contact with cigarette smoke
    b. overeating
    c. lack of exercise
    d. too much exercise
    e. stress

8. People with asthma are better off living in a warm, dry climate, such as that of Arizona.

    True                False

9. People with asthma can exercise moderately, but they have to avoid too much exertion.

    True                False

10. Asthma causes no permanent lung damage.

    True                False

11. Asthma can be cured with some of the new medications now available.

    True                False

12. Children with asthma tend to have a common psychological profile: fearful, unathletic, and overly attached to their parents.

    True                False

13. Which, if any, of the following environmental factors are likely to trigger an asthma attack?
    a. a new carpet
    b. an air conditioner
    c. a dehumidifier
    d. the strong odor of perfume
    e. pollen on a dry, windy day in the fall

14. Which, if any, of the following items are helpful in preventing asthma attacks?
    a. vinyl or plastic covering for furniture
    b. an air conditioner
    c. a dehumidifier
    d. well-insulated, double-glazed windows
    e. a vacuum cleaner

15. How has the asthma death rate changed since 1978?
    a. decreased by half
    b. decreased by 10 percent
    c. stayed the same
    d. risen 10 percent
    e. doubled

Ready? Here are the answers, with explanations. How much did you know about this widespread disease?

1. Asthma is primarily psychological in origin. When a person has eliminated stress in life, asthma tends to disappear.    *False*

Asthma is a genuine organic condition in which the lungs become chronically inflamed, and as a result, are overly sensitive to many internal and external factors: allergens and irritants such as dust, animal dander, mold, foods and food additives, wood smoke, chemical fumes, cold air, and a wide range of other substances, some known and some as yet unknown. Stress may be one of these factors; certainly, there are documented instances of people having an asthma attack in response to a stressful situation. However, these people already had asthma. Stress did not *cause* the asthma—it merely triggered an asthma attack. A person without asthma might have responded to the same stress with a headache, a stomachache, excessive fatigue, a sore neck, or any number of other physical responses. A person with asthma might respond in the same ways—or he or she might have an asthma attack. (For more on the relationship between asthma and stress, see Chapter 8.)

2. Most children who have asthma outgrow the disease by adulthood.    *False*

For the children and their parents who are waiting for this disease to be "outgrown," this may be one of the cruelest myths around. Half of all children who have had asthma go on to experience symptoms even in their teenage years. And about half have gotten to the point of having no symptoms by age fifteen. However, those who are apparently "symptom-free" are only in remission. Their symptoms might easily recur in adulthood, especially if the disease hasn't been properly treated, or if their allergies continue untreated. (For more on childhood asthma, see Chapter 13.)

3. There are two basic types of asthma: *intrinsic,* caused by internal biological factors, and *extrinsic,* caused by reactions to allergens and environmental factors.    *False*

Until recently, doctors generally believed in this way of classifying asthma, and you may still encounter many doctors who use these categories. The latest research, however, suggests that the terms "intrinsic" and "extrinsic" aren't really very helpful. First, no one really knows what causes intrinsic asthma; it's more or less defined as anything that *isn't* extrinsic asthma (although asthma is clearly related to allergy), leading many experts to suspect that at least some intrinsic asthma is triggered by external causes that we simply haven't identified yet. Second, a person may experience both intrinsic and extrinsic asthma, so the categories don't really help doctors to determine any particular course of treatment. Despite the fact that asthma is so widespread, we really know remarkably little about what causes it. In addition, other conditions have symptoms that are similar to asthma, and the many types of asthma may look quite different from one another. (For more on the various types of asthma, see Chapter 3.)

4. You are at increased risk of getting asthma if someone in your family has it.   *True*

Asthma's characteristic of clustering within families leads many scientists to believe that the disease has a genetic origin. On the other hand, the incidence of asthma has risen dramatically in the past twenty years—a period far too short to reflect any significant changes in the gene pool. Only 6.5 percent of families in which neither parent has asthma have a child with asthma, whereas close to 28 percent of families in which one parent has asthma have a child who has asthma. Among families in which both parents have asthma, over 63 percent have at least one child with asthma. The more blood relatives with asthma a child has, the more likely that child is to develop asthma.

Put another way, when compared with children whose parents do not have asthma, children with one parent who has asthma are three to six times likelier to develop the disease, and children with two parents who have asthma are ten times more at risk. Likewise, identical twins, who come from the same genetic material (one egg fertilized by a single sperm), are more likely to share allergies than are fraternal twins (who come from two separate fertilized eggs), and allergies seem to be related to asthma.

The very latest thinking about asthma suggests that a genetic predisposition is part of the picture. Diseases such as Down's syndrome are completely determined by genetic problems; asthma, by contrast, may be more like obesity, reflecting a combination of genetic, environmental, and behavioral factors. In other words, the genetic material that you were born with, the amount of asthma-causing factors in your environment, and your lifestyle would all somehow combine to put you more or less at risk for asthma. In that scenario, your genetic makeup is one element that might lead you to develop asthma—but only one element. (For more on the causes of asthma, see Chapter 3.)

5. You are far more likely to develop asthma if you live with someone (e.g., a spouse or a roommate) who has the disease.     *False*

Asthma is *not* contagious. Being around someone with asthma will not put you at risk in any way if you yourself do not have asthma. Likewise, a child without asthma has nothing to fear from a child who has asthma.

6. Which, if any, of the following factors is likely to cause people to develop asthma?     *a. smoking; c. lack of exercise; d. too much exercise*

Doctors used to believe that virtually all asthma developed in childhood. However, adult-onset asthma is becoming commonly recognized. It's possible that in some cases, adults with this type of asthma had asthma as children and their symptoms were either misdiagnosed as bronchitis or as other types of infections or simply never diagnosed at all. In other cases, the asthma may genuinely appear for the first time sometime after age twenty. Either way, a latent tendency to asthma can certainly be triggered by smoking, which irritates the airways.

It's not exactly accurate to say that lack of exercise causes asthma, but people who don't exercise *are* likely to have less lung capacity than those who do, putting them more at risk for asthma if other asthma-causing factors (allergens, environmental pollutants, a genetic tendency toward the disease) are already present. On the other hand, vigorous exercise can actually trigger asthma in some people—though again, only if a predisposition to the disease is already present. (For more on asthma and exercise, see Chapter 9.)

7. Which, if any, of the following factors is likely to trigger an asthma attack in a person who has already had at least one

asthma attack?   *a. contact with cigarette smoke; d. too much exercise; e. stress*

Any way you look at it, cigarette smoke is generally bad for people with asthma. If you or someone you live with has asthma, the single best thing you can do for yourself or your loved one is to *stop smoking.* For some people, even coming into a room where someone had been smoking a few hours ago can trigger an asthma attack, and any kind of contact with cigarette smoke can interfere with ciliary activity in the airways.

Regular exercise can be of enormous benefit to the person with asthma, but failure to exercise won't actually bring on an attack. However, too much exercise or exercise done without properly warming up can trigger an attack, as can exercise done in polluted air, such as jogging on a busy street during rush hour. Stress can also trigger an attack in some cases. Overeating may be a problem for other reasons, but it won't trigger an asthma attack unless the person eats something to which he or she has an adverse reaction. (For more on asthma and exercise, see Chapter 9.)

8. People with asthma are better off living in a warm, dry climate, such as that of Arizona.   *False*

For years, people with asthma believed that moving to the desert would solve their breathing problems–but no such luck. Warm, dry climates breed weeds and grasses, exposing the asthma sufferer to a wide variety of pollens that may be just as irritating as urban pollution and cold weather. Some asthma sufferers may respond well to certain environments, and you personally may find Arizona to be your promised land. But before making a permanent move in order to solve your asthma or allergy problems, first live in your new locale for a full year to find out if you have allergic reactions to local pollens or molds that might appear only in a particular season. Even so, about half of those who move in order to escape a particular allergen wind up developing a brand-new allergy to some element indigenous to their new location. For people with these external and unavoidable allergies, immunotherapy (allergy shots) can help to decrease the level of sensitivity. (For more on asthma and the environment, see Chapter 6.)

9. People with asthma can exercise moderately, but they have to avoid too much exertion.   *False*

As mentioned before, asthma can sometimes be triggered–not caused–by certain types of exercise. However, some Olympic Gold Medalists have asthma, and they clearly have exerted their systems to an extent far beyond anything that the rest of us might undertake. If you understand your body and its limits, you can certainly exercise vigorously–as long as you follow a few reasonable precautions. (For more on exercise, see Chapter 9.)

10. Asthma causes no permanent lung damage.   *False*

Doctors used to believe that the effects of asthma were entirely reversible. Now we're not so sure. Formerly, we thought that asthma attacks occurred when the bronchial muscles, the muscles that surround the airways, spasmodically contracted and constricted the airways–a process known as *bronchospasm*–and that with proper medication, these muscles could be made to relax and dilate, or widen. Thus, if an asthma attack were controlled with *bronchodilators*–medications that make the airways dilate–the damage caused by asthma could be reversed.

Now, however, we know that asthma includes an underlying chronic condition: inflamed, hyperresponsive lungs. The basement membrane, or lining beneath the mucous layer (mucosa) in the airways, becomes thickened, and many cells accumulate in the mucosa. If the inflammation continues over a long enough period and is not properly treated, the process becomes less reversible.

The good news is that it is usually possible to bring asthma under control and to enjoy good health. The person who follows the recommendations in this book–living a healthy lifestyle that includes avoiding known allergens, maintaining a nutritious diet, getting appropriate exercise, having a good attitude, and using medication appropriately–can go from being someone who has been hospitalized several times with severe attacks to someone who leads a "normal," healthy, vigorous life.

11.  Asthma can be cured with some of the new medications now available.  *False*

Like many other chronic conditions, asthma can be managed, or controlled. However, it cannot yet be cured. If you have asthma, your lungs have a tendency to be overly sensitive to certain stimuli, and so far, we know of no medication or lifestyle change that can completely remove that tendency. The good news is that there is a great deal that you can do to lessen that tendency to the point where you feel great, engage in the activities you enjoy, and face life free of the constant fear of an asthma attack.

12.  Children with asthma tend to have a common psychological profile: fearful, unathletic, and overly attached to their parents.  *False*

This myth about children with asthma has its roots in two related ideas, one true and one false. The false idea is that asthma is primarily a psychological problem, one that fearful children develop or that overprotective parents evoke. In fact, all sorts of children with all sorts of parents have asthma. Likewise, many fearful children with overprotective parents do not have asthma.

However, children with asthma may become fearful. Not being able to breathe is a terrifying experience, and a child who is not helped to cope with that fear may indeed extend his or her anxiety to many other areas of life. Also, it would be hard to conceive of a parent who, after taking a child to the emergency room or watching that child struggle to breathe, did not feel at least somewhat anxious and fearful on that child's behalf. Coping with your natural responses to the terrifying experience of an asthma attack is an enormous challenge, whether you're the child experiencing the attack or the parent watching it.

Exercise can trigger asthma attacks or symptoms. Some children experience difficulty in breathing and have chest pains and other asthma symptoms when they exercise and, because their problem is never diagnosed, simply avoid exercise. (Some experts recommend that any child who avoids exercise or who suddenly stops exercising be tested for asthma, even if he or she has no other symptoms.) Other children understand that exercise can bring on an asthma attack and, without the proper support of parents or coaches, simply stop exercising. With the right kind of help, however, most of these children could certainly be just as athletic as their classmates who do not have asthma. In any case, an aversion to exercise does not cause asthma. (For more on asthma and children, see Chapter 13.)

13. Which, if any, of the following environmental factors are likely to trigger an asthma attack?   *a. a new carpet;   b. an air conditioner;   c. a dehumidifier;   d. the strong odor of perfumes;   e. pollen on a dry, windy day in the fall*

Some new carpets are likely to give off chemical fumes that can trigger an asthma attack. Air conditioners are usually helpful, but if filters are not cleaned regularly, the fan may spread dust through the indoor air. A dehumidifier will help control humidity, but if it has a reservoir with standing water, it can be a prime breeding ground for mold, which is then circulated throughout the house, potentially triggering attacks. Strong smells, including that of perfumes, can also sometimes bring on an attack.

People who are allergic to pollens may find that their asthma worsens during pollen season, particularly if they spend a great deal of time outdoors. Plants such as ragweed pollinate in the fall, trees pollinate in the spring, and grasses pollinate in the late spring and summer. These all can cause allergic reactions and trigger asthma attacks in sensitive people, and these all are widespread throughout the United States.

14. Which, if any, of the following items are helpful in preventing asthma attacks?   *a. vinyl or plastic covering for furniture;   b. an air conditioner;   c. a dehumidifier;   d. a vacuum cleaner*

Upholstered furniture can collect or generate dust, which is a powerful trigger for many people with asthma. Impermeable coverings are easier to keep dust-free. Leather furniture is less permeable, less likely to contain dust mites and molds.

Properly cleaned and fitted with the right filters, an air conditioner can help keep air clean; otherwise, like the dehumidifier, it can be a breeding ground for mold. A dehumidifier that is kept clean and mold-free can help some people with asthma, because keeping indoor air at less than 50 percent humidity helps inhibit the growth of dust mites and molds.

Regular use of a vacuum cleaner fitted with a HEPA filter can cut down on dust—but some vacuum cleaners can actually stir up dust, which in turn might trigger an asthma attack. (For more on how to purify the indoor environment, see Chapter 6.)

15. How has the asthma death rate changed since 1978?
*doubled*

According to the National Bureau of Health Statistics, the death toll from asthma has nearly doubled since 1978, to some five thousand deaths a year in the United States alone. Not only is asthma becoming more widespread, it is also becoming more severe and more likely to cause either hospitalization or death. (For more on why this might be happening, see Chapter 2.)

Why are the myths about asthma so prevalent? And why are the facts so little understood?

One reason is that scientific knowledge is changing very rapidly. We now know a great deal more about asthma than we knew ten or even five years ago. This new knowledge has led to new medications and new therapy.

We also still have a lot to learn about asthma. Although most doctors and health care providers who treat asthma are generally hopeful about the good results that their patients can achieve, they also have a lot of questions. They don't always know why a particular course of treatment works—only that it does. In an atmosphere of exploration and discovery, it can be hard to separate facts from myths.

Two things, however, are certain: One, asthma has become an increasingly serious problem, affecting more people and affecting them more seriously than ever before. (For more on the spread of asthma, see Chapter 2.) And two, by using the approaches described in this book and by working with your doctor, a person with asthma can control the disease and can lead a happy, productive, energetic life.

# 2

# The Way *Your* Asthma Works:

## *How Your Body Reacts, the Different Kinds, and Diagnosis*

One day, Angela is walking home from her bus stop, and a bus passes by, releasing a huge cloud of exhaust. It's a cold February evening, and Angela has been fighting a cold all week, so her nose is stuffed up and her chest feels congested. Suddenly, she finds herself gasping and wheezing for breath. Angela stops to catch her breath, but the more cold air she pulls into her lungs, the more difficulty she has in breathing. Her nose is completely clogged with mucus, which she now feels dripping back into her throat as well. Her chest hurts, and the harder she works to breathe through her mouth, the more her chest seems to tighten up. Angela starts to cough, which makes things even worse, because she can't catch her breath between coughs. Somehow, she manages to stagger into a nearby store, still coughing and gasping. After a few minutes in the warm air of the store, she feels a little better, but her chest still hurts, her lungs feel raw, and her throat is sore. In addition, Angela is very, very scared. While the episode lasted, she really felt that she might suffocate, choking on her own mucus and unable to get control of her breath. She calls a taxi to take her home, and when she gets home, she calls her doctor right away.

Angela's first asthma attack was triggered by cold air and bus exhaust. But when Angela's doctor sees her, he will probably explain that Angela had been developing asthma for a long time. All during the winter, when Angela had been getting bronchitis and had been heavily exposed to dust mites, her airways were gradually becoming inflamed. The inflammation was narrowing the airways through which she breathed, while both her infections and her growing asthma were leading her body to produce excess mucus. Angela had developed asthma.

Because Angela had acquired this underlying condition, she was susceptible to an asthma trigger, a factor in her environment or her diet that might set off an asthma attack. In Angela's case, there were two triggers: the cold, dry air of winter and the exhaust fumes of the passing bus. These two factors did not cause Angela's asthma; they only caused her asthma attack. A person without asthma walking by Angela's side would also have breathed in the cold air and the bus exhaust, but he or she would not have had an asthma attack.

## What Is Asthma and What Causes It?

Asthma is a long-term chronic condition marked by four basic abnormalities in the lungs:

1. The airways are narrowed.
2. The airways are inflamed.
3. The lungs secrete excess mucus.
4. The airways are overly responsive to a variety of triggers, including allergens, infections, irritants, exercise, certain medications, and dry, cold air.

No one knows what causes asthma. Other conditions mimic or aggravate bronchospasm: bronchitis or emphysema, or the somewhat less common bronchopulmonary aspergillosis, congestive heart failure, chronic infectious bronchitis resulting from cystic fibrosis, ciliary dysfunction syndrome, upper airway obstruction, pertussis syndrome, psychogenic coughs, bronchiolitis obliterans, chronic eosinophilic pneumonia, paradoxical vocal cord dysfunction, or vasculitides.

Until recently, explanations of asthma focused on the activity within the lungs and the airways. The word used most often was bronchoconstriction—the constriction, or tightening up, of the bronchial system, the muscles surrounding the airways. As a result, treatment focused on bronchodilation, getting the bronchial muscles around the airways to relax so that the airways could dilate, or open up. Inhalers contained bronchodilators, medication that caused the muscles to relax and the airways to expand. A person with asthma who felt an attack coming on was urged to expand his or her airways by inhaling a bronchodilator.

## *Extrinsic vs. Intrinsic Asthma*

When scientists viewed asthma in this way, they divided asthma into extrinsic asthma (triggered by a foreign substance entering the lungs) and intrinsic asthma (triggered by some mysterious process that no one really understood). As mentioned in Chapter 1, however, this division has fallen out of favor, partly because doctors suspect that much intrinsic asthma was triggered by a foreign substance that was simply not identified, partly because many individuals seemed to have both types of asthma, and partly because the mystery surrounding intrinsic asthma was not very satisfying. After all, why should the bronchial muscles around the lungs simply contract by themselves, for no apparent reason?

## *Asthma: An Allergic Disease*

The latest research suggests that asthma may be the result of a disordered immune response leading to release of mediators (chemical molecules) by cells in the airways. In this view, asthma is a disorder in which the body is on a kind of permanent red alert, reacting and overreacting to a wide variety of factors in the environment. The body's violent reactions extend to factors that aren't actually dangerous, such as dust mites and cold air, as well as to factors that may be dangerous, such as pollution and certain organisms such as viruses or mycoplasma. Thus, what used to be called intrinsic asthma would be explained as the body reacting to a perceived threat of some kind.

Regardless of what triggers an asthma attack, the body's "cure" is worse than the disease. Trying to deal with what it perceives as a dangerous foreign substance, the body goes into an asthmatic reaction that may well prove deadlier than the dust mite or pollen that provoked the reaction in the first place. In an asthma attack, the body is literally harassing itself, even as it tries to attack the "foreign invader" that it fears. The airways are suffering from chronic inflammation that has left them swollen, narrowed, and so sensitive that a wide variety of triggers can make them contract, as the lung tissues swell and fill with mucus. The attack is the result of an underlying problem: the chronic inflammation of the lungs.

This is why many doctors now view the constant use of bronchodilators as a problem, for they masked a dangerous underlying condition even as they treated the symptoms of that condition. A person with asthma might rely on a bronchodilator to open up the airways, even as the lungs are becoming more and more inflamed. The more inflamed the lungs became, the more constricted the airways became, and the more medication was needed to make them dilate. The person with asthma might find himself or herself using an inhaler more and more frequently, as the bronchodilation lasted for shorter and shorter periods. Finally, one day, the bronchodilator might be unable to push the exhausted airways into expanding. And the person with asthma would suddenly be left to experience the full effect of years of inflammation—and would probably be rushed to a hospital with difficulty breathing.

## **Healthy Breathing**

Take a deep breath. Notice the way that the air moves through your nose and mouth, down through your throat, into your chest, and deep into your diaphragm. If you had croup, you would feel an obstruction high up in your airways, where your vocal cords are, in the back of your throat. (Croup is a condition marked by swollen vocal cords.) If you had emphysema, you would have an obstruction lower down in your airways, closer to the diaphragm, which would indicate that much of the delicate tissue through which oxygen passes had already been destroyed. If you have asthma, however, you might not notice any obstruction—unless you are having an attack. Then you would be suffering from an obstruction in the middle of your chest, where the small airways are.

### *A Unique Process*

Breathing is unique among our vital processes: it's the only activity that we both do unconsciously and are able to control to some extent. Your heart beats without your choosing it, and unless you've been engaged in esoteric types of meditation, you won't feel able to slow your heartbeat or speed it up by a conscious act of will. You also won't be able to choose your own blood pressure, which indicates the force at which your blood is rushing through your body. On the other hand, eating, which is as necessary to life as a heartbeat, is a wholly conscious activity. You choose when to eat, and you see yourself as being fully in control of the muscle movements that bring the food into your mouth. You have remarkably little to do with digestion, which happens "on its own."

Breathing is the only act that happens on its own but which you can learn to control relatively easily. You can choose to breathe deeply or shallowly, quickly or slowly. Yet, most of the time, most people are as unaware of their breathing as they are of their heartbeat or their digestion.

A person having an asthma attack, however, is wholly focused on breathing. Ironically, this means that people with asthma have gotten to know this vital process at its worst, when it is working least well and being done least effectively. So a good first step in understanding asthma is understanding the process of healthy breathing.

The purpose of breathing is to take air out of the environment and put it into your body, so that the oxygen from that air can be used by every single one of your cells. Here's what's involved in taking a breath:

1. Air is pulled through the nose into the nasal passages, where it is warmed, humidified, and cleaned by tiny hairs (ciliated cells).

2. The air passes through the pharynx (throat) and the larynx (voice box) into the trachea (windpipe).

3. Below the upper part of the breastbone, the trachea divides into two passages, the mainstem bronchi–specifically, the right mainstem bronchus and the left mainstem bronchus. The right bronchus carries air to and from the right lung; the left bronchus does the same with the left lung. (Airway is another word for bronchus.)

4. After a few inches, each mainstem bronchus divides into smaller bronchi, which in turn divide into still smaller bronchi, and on and on and on until the bronchi have divided into very tiny airways known as *bronchioles*.

5. As the airways become progressively narrower, the air passing through them moves faster. (Think of squeezing a toothpaste tube. The tighter you squeeze the tube, the narrower it becomes, and the faster the toothpaste moves through it.)

6. The bronchioles lead into about 300 million evenly distributed air sacs called *alveoli*. The alveoli are tiny globes of lung tissue wrapped in *capillaries*, which are tiny blood vessels.

7. The alveoli absorb air and extract the oxygen from it.

8. While the alveoli are extracting oxygen, they are also releasing carbon dioxide, a waste product that your body doesn't need and that you will eventually exhale. This exchange of gases with the environment–taking in oxygen and giving off carbon dioxide–is called respiration.

9. The alveoli transmit the oxygen into the neighboring capillaries. Technically, the oxygen atoms in the lungs react with the hemoglobin in the blood, creating oxyhemoglobin–oxygen in the bloodstream.

10. The oxyhemoglobin is carried from the capillaries into the pulmonary veins and thus into the heart, which then pumps it through the arteries, transporting it throughout

the body. Delivering the oxygen, of course, is the purpose of the whole exercise, because every cell in the body needs oxygen to function properly.

Are you impressed with the aerodynamic efficiency of this miraculous mechanism? You should be, for it involves a whole system of chemical messengers and muscles that continually work together to keep your body functioning. Take another deep breath, noticing every part of your body that was involved. If you had total body awareness, here's what you would have felt as you inhaled:

- Your nostril muscles contracted.
- Your vertebral column, or spine, extended.
- Your neck muscles contracted.
- Your first rib moved upward.
- The muscles of your internal diaphragm (the area just below your ribs) contracted, moving your ribs back down.
- Your stomach muscles contracted.

And while all this was going on, here's what was happening inside your respiratory system, which involves both your lungs and your brain:

- Fluid was being sucked into your capillaries from the space between the layers of tissue that line your lungs.
- Oxygen was passing into your capillaries and combining with red blood cells—that oxyhemoglobin mentioned earlier.
- Your brain was monitoring levels of oxygen in your blood and sending out updates to your lungs. Thus, if you had been running in place for two minutes before you did this exercise, you would probably find yourself breathing faster and more deeply. That's because your brain would have realized that oxygen had been used up by the exercise. As

a result, your brain would tell your lungs to work harder for a little while to replace the lost oxygen.

Chapter 9 offers specific breathing exercises: some for everyday practice; others to mitigate an asthma attack.

## Inflammation and Constriction

Now let's look at how asthma interrupts and upsets the breathing process. Recall that the small bronchi (airways) and bronchioles are where asthma strikes. When these portions of the lungs become inflamed, the breathing process is disrupted.

Inflammation is a response from the immune system. It is your body's way of responding to a substance not normally found in your body, a substance that your body perceives as toxic, or harmful. For example, suppose that a bee stings you. If you are allergic, as the venom from the bee enters through your skin, immune cells from the surrounding tissue and from your bloodstream rush to the site of the sting. If you are allergic, the immunoglobulin E on the surface of the cells causes the cells to release chemicals into the area. The *inflammatory response* that results from all this chemical activity includes three components:

1. Swelling—perhaps just around the site of the sting, perhaps a wider area, depending on how aggressively your immune system responds to the bee venom protein.
2. Pain—because the chemicals released by your immune system as well as the chemicals released by the bee affect the nerves in the area.
3. Redness—because both the venom and the immune system cause blood vessels in the area to swell.

Now picture this response taking place within your lungs. Suppose you have asthma and you inhale a substance that your body perceives as a toxin—perhaps a real toxin such as cigarette smoke or bus exhaust; perhaps a harmless substance such as household dust or pollen. Your immune system goes into high gear, and the bronchial lining—the tissues that line the airways—become inflamed. In other words, they swell and turn red. You don't actually feel pain in your lungs, however, because bronchial lining has no pain receptors in it. What does happen is that the swelling and bronchoconstriction due to the inflammatory response tend to narrow the passageways through which air travels.

Inflammation has another effect: it makes the airways hyperresponsive, or supersensitive, to events that they might normally ignore. In other words, a normal lung would ignore a speck of pollen or a grain of house dust, but a hyperresponsive asthmatic lung might react vigorously to this perceived insult. The airways are meant to be dynamic structures that can change size and behavior in response to the body's need for oxygen. When the airways are inflamed and hyperresponsive, they tend to contract far too much, a process known as bronchospasm.

Inflammation also produces excess mucus, as Angela discovered. All lungs contain goblet cells, located in the airway walls, whose job is to keep the airways "oiled" with mucus. When an airway is inflamed, however, the goblet cells produce far too much mucus—so much that the airways can become clogged.

Another part of the inflammation process is known as mucosal edema. This *edema,* or swelling, further narrows the airways.

### *The Process of Inflammation*

1. The body experiences an "invasion" from an allergen or irritant.
2. The immune system responds to the invasion with a complex series of chemical reactions known as the inflammatory cascade (for more detail on these reactions, see Chapter 4). The inflammatory cascade is part of the body's immune system, whose job is to destroy "foreign invaders."
3. Cells such as eosingshils and neutroplasts are attracted to the area, and while trying to destroy the "invader" the inflammatory cascade also destroys some of the tissue lining the airways. That's because it "thinks" that the invader might be hiding in that tissue.

4. The tissue lining the airways becomes swollen. Because the swollen tissue takes up so much room, air can't move through the airways as quickly as it should.

5. The goblet cells release gobs of mucus to protect the raw and irritated inflamed tissue—but the excess mucus also blocks the airways, which then have trouble transmitting enough oxygen into the bloodstream.

6. Meanwhile, the irritated nerves surrounding the airways signal the muscles that surround the bronchial tubes, which then constrict. Chemicals known as leukotriens produced by cells that have moved into the area also cause smooth-muscle constriction. This is the process known as bronchospasm. Now the airways are not only inflamed and swollen on the inside, they are also constricted from pressure of the muscles that surround them.

7. The person with asthma experiences wheezing, shortness of breath, coughing, excess phlegm, and tightness in the chest.

## Asthma Attacks

If you've never had an asthma attack, here's a way to find out what it feels like. Put a small straw in your mouth and pinch your nose shut, so that you can breathe only through the straw in your mouth. For extra realism, try climbing a flight of stairs, lifting something heavy, or even talking—with only the tiny amount of air you can get through the straw. Of course, one major difference is that you have control over this experiment; you can make it stop. Another major difference is that you know how bad it's going to get, so you don't have to experience the overwhelming panic that most people with asthma feel during an attack. (If you or your child has asthma and you're trying to convey to loved ones, co-workers, or teachers what it feels like, you might urge them to try this experiment.)

## Catching Your Breath

During the early part of an asthma attack, the swelling and mucus don't block air from coming into the lungs. Rather, they block air from going out; they prevent the person with asthma from exhaling normally. A person who has very severe asthma with highly swollen airways and overfilled lungs, may also have difficulty inhaling.

Because Angela was only experiencing her first attack, she was able to pass through it relatively quickly, without the aid of medication. If she were to continue to experience such attacks without receiving the proper treatment, she would soon have trouble inhaling as well as exhaling. At that point, she would be working extra hard just to breathe, because her airways would have become so narrow that her bronchial muscles and many other supplementary muscles would all be working overtime just to move air in and out.

### *When Asthma Threatens Life*

When the airways have narrowed to this extent, asthma becomes truly dangerous. When you have to work so hard just to breathe, you are in danger of finally becoming too tired to push air through the airways. Then the body won't receive enough oxygen, and your life will be threatened.

Like most chronic diseases, each aspect of asthma tends to make the other aspects worse. For example, breathing was designed to be done through the nose, so that the nasal passages can warm, purify, and humidify the air that passes through. But if mucus is plugging your nose, so that you have to breathe through your mouth, the air going into your lungs is dry, dusty, and cool—and far more likely to irritate sensitive airway linings.

Moreover, if the airway linings are already irritated, the air entering the lungs encounters uneven, swollen, inflamed surfaces, not the smooth passageways that nature intended. These uneven surfaces move the air along less efficiently, with less speed and less pressure. Airway resistance to the entering air can be up to twenty-five times greater than normal. Imagine how much harder the bronchial muscles have to work under these circumstances.

Meeting such resistance, the lungs compensate by overinflating. Imagine running in place for two minutes. Think of how far your lungs would be inflating at the end of that exercise. Now notice how much less they are inflating as you sit quietly, reading this book. Imagine that just sitting here, reading, took as much work from your lungs as running in place. You can easily see how asthma causes the lungs to work overtime and how your chest muscles are being put under an extra strain.

### *A Total Effect*

If the body receives less oxygen than it needs, the function of every cell in the body is impaired. So if you have asthma, your entire body is trying to compensate for the times during an attack when you're not getting enough oxygen.

In this way, asthma is different from other chronic diseases. On the most basic level, we need to take in oxygen with every breath. And when a person has active asthma, every breath is work. You can't take a break, you can't rest for a while. You have to keep breathing, in and out, in and out, every few seconds. Yet during an attack, or when you've suffered from asthma for a long time, every breath seems to take an enormous effort. You don't even get time off when you're asleep. Imagine the strain on your entire system, the cost to your energy, to the nutrients you've stored, to your overall resistance to disease and stress. No wonder that even Angela, who is just beginning to experience asthma, feels chronically exhausted, depleted, and susceptible to infection!

But remember that this process is reversible. It is possible to restore your energy and soothe your immune system by identifying and avoiding allergens; to lower your sensitivity to some allergens with immunotherapy; to try treating infection if it is present in the bronchii or sinuses in order to manage nasal obstruction; and to work *with* your breathing process to prevent and mitigate asthma attacks.

## Components of an Asthma Attack

Because an attack is so overwhelming and frightening, you may have difficulty knowing what's going on in your body at the time. It's helpful to be able to visualize what's happening (and to use breathing exercises, both to improve your breathing and to calm yourself down; see Chapter 9). Here are some of the major elements of an asthma attack:

*Wheezing* This sound reflects blockage in various airways: within the bronchioles, or between the larynx and bronchioles. There are lots of reasons for wheezing, of course, many of which are not due to asthma. In asthma, however, wheezing results from the way that the airways and muscles "swell" during bronchospasm, which blocks the airways. The blockage happens only during the time you exhale. Wheezing can be chestwide or local; it can be constant or can come and go; it can appear in a pattern or apparently at random. Sometimes the lungs may be inflamed but not blocked, so there is no wheezing. Alternatively, the lungs may be so thoroughly blocked, with mucus, swelling, or both, that no sound gets through at all.

*Coughing* A cough is how the body helps us get rid of material that blocks our airways. It may be a nerve reflex–that is, involuntary–or it may be voluntary, as when you decide to clear your throat. Technically, a cough begins with inspiration (breathing in) and is followed by a closing of the *glottis* (the elongated space between the vocal cords) during expiration (breathing out). The buildup of pressure in the lungs, followed by a sudden opening of the glottis, produces a burst of air, which we know as a cough.

Coughing during an asthma attack is usually the attempt of the lungs to remove the buildup of mucus, which, as mentioned earlier, is secreted in excessive quantities during an attack. Normally, *cilia*–little hairs that line the lungs, picking up dust and other particles–keep the lungs free of foreign objects, but if there's too much mucus (or too much of something else, such as smoke) in the lungs, the cilia aren't enough to do the job, and coughing is also needed. In medical terms, a productive cough helps expel mucus, while a nonproductive cough doesn't bring up anything.

During an asthma attack, you may be seized by a fit of nonproductive coughing, in which the lungs try desperately to expel the built-up mucus, but fail. The mucus may be too thick because you are dehydrated at this point, or there may simply be too much mucus. On the other hand, you may feel like coughing but not be able to because the airways are too obstructed.

*Shortness of Breath* Also known as *dyspnea,* this is the result of not being able to exhale properly. If you can't fully exhale, it's hard to fully inhale.

*Chest Pain* The entire process of an asthma attack puts an enormous strain on the chest muscles, as well as on the back and shoulders. Because all sorts of muscles get involved in the breathing process, you may experience some chest pain during an attack or at other times. Naturally, because chest pain is also a symptom of so many other ailments, you should always report such pain to your doctor. Sudden severe pain during an attack may occur because of a "blowout" of a bleb (a small blister or bubble) and the entry of air into the space outside the immediate lung covering.

*Rapid Breathing* Also known as *tachypnea,* this is a response of many people with asthma to compensate for the blockage in their lungs. Unable to breathe deeply enough because of airway obstruction, you may breathe shallowly but rapidly, to allow more air to pass in and out of the lungs.

*Fatigue* The process of continuing to breathe during an attack is so exhausting that you may experience fatigue as the attack wears on. This is a significant danger sign, as it means you are becoming too tired to breathe.

*Inflated Chest* Because the air is trapped in the lungs during an attack, unable to be properly expelled, the lungs expand, ballooning out with all that trapped air. The chest becomes more crowded, and widens from front to back. At the same time, the diaphram is forced down. Ironically, this response makes it even more difficult to return breathing to normal. (That's why the breathing exercises in Chapter 9 are so important.)

*Speech Problems*  If you can't catch your breath, you can't talk. A person who is experiencing a severe asthma attack will probably speak as little as possible or in short phrases, pausing between each to take a breath.

*Dehydration*  Rapid breathing causes the body to lose water. Having a fever secondary to infection during an asthma attack will also cause dehydration, which in turn can make mucus problems worse. (This is one reason why it's so important for people with asthma to drink lots of water or other fluids. See Chapter 8.)

*Nasal Problems*  Because air comes through the nose, and because the airways connect the nose with the lungs, people with asthma often have nasal problems, which both cause and are affected by the asthma. Allergic reactions frequently cause symptoms in the nose and the airways. Rhinitis (excess secretions from the nose) means that extra mucus may be dripping down into the posterior pharynx, particularly at night. This extra mucus might cause breathing difficulties that actually set off an attack, or it may simply make an attack more painful. Sinusitis (excess secretions from the sinuses) plays a similar role. People with asthma, especially if they are sensitive to aspirin, often have nasal polyps, which interfere with breathing and may have to be medically treated or surgically removed. These are the people who are more likely to be sensitive to aspirin and nonsteroidal medications such as ibuprofen.

## "Do I Have Asthma?"

At this point, you may be wondering whether or not you even have asthma. You may recognize some of the processes we have described, or you may feel that your own case is different. You may also have realized that asthma may be a subtle disease as well as an obvious one, a disease that it's possible to have for some time without realizing it.

Of course, any final diagnosis of asthma should be done by a qualified physician. To help you develop your own awareness, however, we offer these asthma indicators:

### *The Six Warning Signs of Asthma*

1. Are you breathing properly, using the muscles of your diaphragm? Or do you use several accessory muscles to breathe, lifting your shoulders and overworking your chest? A person who is compensating for breathing difficulties caused by asthma may have a "hunched" look, with permanently lifted shoulders and a concave chest.

2. Can you complete a fairly long sentence without drawing an extra breath? If not, your shortness of breath may be caused by asthma-related breathing problems.

3. Do you have a rapid pulse? Of course, many things may speed up a pulse, including caffeine, medications, and anxiety. But not having enough oxygen will also make your pulse race, just as it does when you've been exercising vigorously and using up oxygen.

4. Do you wheeze audibly? Is your breathing heavy and raspy or light and mild? If mucus plugs are blocking your airways, you will probably wheeze—and you may have asthma.

5. Are you frequently anxious? Not being able to breathe is probably the most frightening experience known to humankind. If you have to struggle to breathe, your emotions as well as your lungs are probably engaged in the battle.

6. Do you have pain in your abdomen, back, or breastbone? Are your ribs tender? You may be putting too much strain on your chest, back, and stomach muscles as you try to breathe.

If you experience even three of these six symptoms, you are probably suffering from asthma or some other lung disease. We urge you to discuss these symptoms with your physician and work to treat your condition.

## Getting Tested

If you and your doctor do explore your condition after taking your medical history, there are a number of tests that he or she is likely to order. Here are some of the most common:

*Pulmonary Function Tests (PFTs)* The more elaborate forms of these tests are performed in laboratories; the simpler versions can be done in a doctor's office. Most such tests are done with a spirometer, a computerized instrument. To use it, you put on nose clips, inhale fully, and then breathe out as hard as possible into a mouthpiece and tube. The spirometer, attached to the tube, measures how much air was in the lungs during exhalation–lung volume measurements–and the speed with which the air is exhaled–ventilation measurements.

*Testing Flow Rate* Tests for asthma are essentially designed to measure the extent to which you can exhale. The first sign of an asthma attack is difficulty with expelling air from the lungs. The rate of exhalation is known as flow rate. You may have a reduced flow rate and no other symptoms. In other words, you might have asthma and not even know it. Measuring your flow rate and seeing if it improves after using a bronchodilator drug, would help determine the presence of the disease.

Flow rate can be measured in a number of different ways. One is *Forced Expiratory Volume (FEV)*, which determines the maximum amount of air that you can exhale in half a second (FEV-0.5) or in one second (FEV-1.0). This test can be done in an office or a laboratory.

Another key test is the *Peak Expiratory Flow Rate (PEFR)*, which measures how fast air can be expelled from the lungs. Your doctor will probably want to initially conduct this test, but you can also measure your own peak flow by using a peak-flow meter.

In fact, regular monitoring of your peak flow is sometimes recommended (see Chapter 10).

*Reversibility Test* Your doctor may also use this test to determine whether you have asthma. You would be given some medication, usually a bronchodilator that will help open the airways. If the flow rates described above show improved performance after you have taken the medication, your lung problems are considered reversible—and you are diagnosed with asthma.

*Other Pulmonary Tests* Here are five less common pulmonary tests that your doctor may order:

- *Functional Residual Capacity (FRC), Residual Volume (RV),* and *Total Lung Capacity (TLC),* all of which measure the air "trapped" in the lungs by asthma.
- *Inspiratory Flow Measurements,* which measure the flow of air as it is breathed in. If you are suffering from blockage of the upper airways, you don't have asthma—remember, asthma occurs when the lower airways are blocked. But your symptoms may be similar to those of someone with asthma; hence, this test.
- *Diffusing Capacity,* which measures your lungs' ability to diffuse oxygen throughout the lung. People with asthma usually show a normal response, so an abnormality on this test might indicate another lung disease, such as emphysema.
- *Arterial Blood Gases (ABG),* a blood test that measures oxygen and carbon dioxide levels in the blood, as well as the acidity of arterial blood. During a mild or moderate asthma attack, blood carbon dioxide levels may be too low. If the process continues and becomes severe, the carbon dioxide will be elevated and the oxygen level will decrease.
- *Percent oxygen saturation* can be measured without drawing blood and is commonly used to follow progress during an attack.

*Provocative Testing* Of course, any of the tests mentioned here may show perfectly normal lung activity—except during an asthma attack. Therefore, your doctor may order provocative testing, in which the tester attempts to provoke an asthma attack and then to measure lung and blood activity while the attack is proceeding. Naturally, such testing should only be done by highly experienced personnel and under closely supervised conditions, in case the attack gets out of hand. The "provocation" might make use of a provocative substance, such as methacholine or histamine, or certain allergens. Or you might be asked to exercise on a bicycle or treadmill.

*Allergy Testing* Because asthma and allergies are intimately related, your doctor may wish to order allergy tests for you. These tests may show what allergen is causing the asthmatic reaction and may lead to avoidance measures that can reduce the inflammation and hyperirritability of the airways. (For more on this type of testing, see Chapter 5.)

*Sweat Test* Sometimes asthma is mimicked by cystic fibrosis, a hereditary disease of the lungs and pancreas that is found mostly in children. The sweat of a child with cystic fibrosis will show a higher concentration of salt than the sweat of a child with asthma. Doctors use this test to decide whether a child has cystic fibrosis. It is possible, however, to have both disorders.

*Complete Blood Count (CBC)* A complete blood count can detect an infection by finding a higher-than-normal white blood cell count. It might also point to allergies by showing increased levels of eosinophils, cells used by the immune system to ward off an "invader." (For more on asthma and allergies, see Chapters 4 and 5.)

*Chest X ray* If you have asthma without complications, your chest X ray will not show it. However, if your symptoms are being caused by another lung problem, your chest X ray may reveal it. Likewise, complications such as pneumonia will show up on an X ray.

*Sinus X ray* Sometimes a sinus X ray can reveal a sinus infection or inflammation, a condition that might aggravate asthma.

Limited CT scans of sinuses cost little more and show the anatomy in much more detail.

*Sputum and Nasal Secretion Examination*   In this test, your doctor examines the phlegm you cough up as well as the secretions from your nose. Some physicians use a small scoop in the nasal passage, and others have you blow to bring secretions to the front of the nose. The doctor is looking for cells indicating active infection and for eosinophils, which would usually indicate allergy.

*Bronchoscopy*   Doctors rarely order this to diagnose asthma, but they may use it to rule out conditions that mimic asthma, such as blockage of the lungs by a foreign body. The test is also used to diagnose asthma complications, such as certain infections. In this procedure, the doctor uses a long, flexible, fiber-optic tube—an endoscope—to directly examine the major airways. Sometimes a bronchoscopy involves taking a small piece of lung tissue for further examination under a microscope. Very occasionally, this procedure is used to remove thick mucus from the lungs in some patients with life-threatening asthma.

*Rhinoscopy*   An endoscope may also be used to examine the interior of the nose and sinuses. A doctor looking for an obstruction in the nose, sinuses, and throat might conduct such a procedure. Nasal polyps are common in patients with asthma. Abnormal closure of the larynx can be demonstrated.

## "What Kind of Asthma Do I Have?"

As mentioned earlier, diagnoses of asthma have changed over the years as doctors have come to understand more about this disease. Here are a few of the most common terms used to describe patterns of symptoms.

*Nocturnal Asthma*   As the name suggests, this means that your asthma gets worse between 2 A.M. and 4 A.M. Doctors speculate that this may occur because mucus can't drain so easily at night. Or it may be in response to allergens in the bedroom, such as the dust mites or fungal spores in the mattress or pillows. Of course, some people with asthma are not allergic, and they may still suffer from nocturnal asthma.

Another theory is that nocturnal asthma occurs as a delayed reaction to some daytime insult. Others have wondered whether an individual's circadian rhythm—the complicated biological clock that regulates sleep, energy levels, and biorhythms—is responsible for nocturnal asthma. It's interesting to note that the hormones epinephrine and cortisol, which help keep the bronchial tubes open, fall to their lowest levels between midnight and 6 A.M., while histamine, a natural chemical that worsens asthma, is at its highest level at night.

Nocturnal asthma leads to loss of sleep and usually indicates uncontrolled asthma.

*Seasonal Asthma* As you might expect, in some people asthma is worse during pollen season. Some studies have linked increased asthma attacks to pollen sources or bursts of mold spores.

*Exercise-induced Asthma* Exercise is a common trigger for many patients with chronic asthma. During exercise, you breathe not only faster but more often through the mouth, causing you to inhale cooler, drier air. As already mentioned, this can irritate the lungs, and inflamed, hyperresponsive lungs might react by setting off an asthma attack. Some patients have asthma only after exercise of four to six minutes. Some note that a combination of exercise and certain foods lead to the symptoms. For more on how to prevent exercise-induced asthma, see Chapter 9. And remember, some Olympic athletes have asthma, so this is a condition that can be overcome by most patients.

*Adult-onset Asthma* As Angela discovered, it is possible to contract asthma as an adult—even in your fifties. Although adult-onset asthma strikes people as early as their late twenties, it poses special challenges to people over age fifty-five. First, adult-onset asthma is harder to diagnose at that age, because congestive heart failure and so-called cardiac asthma (breathing difficulties that result from heart problems rather than from any of the bodily processes described in this chapter) can either mimic or com-

|  | Clinical Features Before Treatment* | |
|---|---|---|
|  | Symptoms† | Nighttime Symptoms |
| Step 4<br>Severe persistent | Continual symptoms<br>Limited physical activity<br>Frequent exacerbations | Frequent |
| Step 3<br>Moderate persistent | Daily symptoms<br>Daily use of inhaled short-acting beta$_2$-agonist<br>Exacerbations affect activity<br>Exacerbations ≥2 times a week; may last days | >1 time a week |
| Step 2<br>Mild persistent | Symptoms >2 times a week but <1 time a day<br>Exacerbations may affect activity | >2 times a month |
| Step 1<br>Mild intermittent | Symptoms ≤2 times a week<br>Asymptomatic and normal PEF between exacerbations<br>Exacerbations brief (from a few hours to a few days); intensity may vary | ≤2 times a month |

*The presence of one of the features of severity is sufficient to place a patient in that category. An individual should be assigned to the most severe grade in which any feature occurs. The characteristics noted in this figure are general and may overlap because asthma is highly variable. Furthermore, an individual's classification may change over time.

†Patients at any level of severity can have mild, moderate, or severe exacerbations. Some patients with intermittent asthma experience severe and life-threatening exacerbations separated by long periods of normal lung function and no symptoms.

(Chart reprinted by permission of Annals of Allergy, Asthma, and Immunology, from Guidelines for Diagnosis and Management of Asthma, Expert Panel Report II, NIH, 1997.)

pound "true" asthma. Asthma can also aggravate coronary heart disease, if the oxygen supplied by the lungs is inadequate for the already-reduced blood supply to the heart. Moreover, the effects of common asthma medications such as theophylline and epinephrine can make heart disease worse; the older classic antihistamines can cause men with enlarged prostates to retain urine;

and oral corticosteroids can worsen the symptoms of glaucoma, cataracts, and osteoporosis.

Older people with asthma should be extra sure to visit their doctors regularly in order to monitor the way in which their asthma interacts with other existing medical conditions. They should work with doctors to explore reduced or alternate medications. They should also make sure that what appear to be the presenting signs of depression—fatigue, sleep disturbances, exhaustion, a general sense of helplessness—are not in fact the body's response to asthma, rather than a psychological problem.

People with arthritis may need special inhalers that are easier to operate. Those with failing eyesight may need color-coded markers to help them read their peak-flow meters. (For more on peak-flow meters, see Chapter 11.) A person who is concerned about forgetfulness may need to make sure all instructions are written down. One who is already taking several medications may need to work out some kind of combination medication with the doctor in order to simplify the treatment program. And of course, all people with asthma should explore pneumonia and flu vaccines with their doctors, because these ailments may set off asthma and other complications.

*Variations of Asthma*   Here is a list of some other "types" of asthma that you may recognize in yourself or in other people. You may have experienced more than one of these triggers of asthma. You may notice certain patterns of symptoms. Or you may have noticed that over the years, you have acquired some new triggers and lost others. These medical terms may no longer be particularly useful, but they may help you to define your own asthma. It's helpful to think of yourself as having your own unique disease with its own special collection of symptoms.

- *Allergic or atopic asthma* is caused by allergies.
- *Cotton-dust asthma, or stripper's asthma, mill fever,* is caused by working with cotton, flax, or hemp.
- *Emphysematous asthma* is emphysema accompanied by asthmatic symptoms.

- *Essential or true asthma* is asthma of unknown cause.
- *Grinder's asthma* is caused by working with grinding metal and inhaling the fine metal particles.
- *Isocyanate asthma* is caused by allergies to toluene diisocyanate, a highly toxic substance used in treating wood and in other industrial processes.
- *Miner's asthma and potter's asthma* are occupational versions of the disease.

### Asthma Patterns You May Encounter

- Asthma with a cough but no wheeze
- Asthma with mucus but without coughing and wheezing
- Moist wheezing with sneezing, runny nose, and other hay fever symptoms
- Exercise-induced asthma
- Cold-air asthma
- Tension in the chest, accompanied by a faint wheeze
- Nighttime tension in the chest
- A sudden, overwhelming flooding with mucus, accompanied by gasping for breath

The classification of asthma as defined by the NAEPP Guidelines report is summaried in the table on page 36. This is helpful in determining types and frequency of medication, evaluations needed, and frequency and type of monitoring and emergency action plans for each patient.

### Two Kinds of Asthma?

The most useful way to approach asthma—for both patients and their doctors—is to do so as individually as possible. People with asthma should keep a journal for at least two weeks, detailing what they notice about their habits, their symptoms, and their feelings. In general, pay close, detailed, respectful attention to your body and to its responses to food, emotion, work, weather, and its environment. Likewise, doctors should approach each patient as individually as possible, seeing him or her as a unique human being rather than as a typical condition or predetermined diagnosis.

That being said, however, it's also useful to conceive of two different categories of asthma. One is primarily driven by allergies and may not even involve chronic inflammation if the exposure to the allergen is short-lived. Attacks of this type of asthma are characterized by an excessive release of mucus or sudden wheezing, and they can usually be attributed to a specific allergen, for example, exposure to cats. This type of asthma would be especially likely to run in families.

The other type of asthma is primarily marked by chronic inflammation of the lungs—which may have been caused by repeated allergic reactions (e.g., living with a cat in the house), but which also may have been caused by occupational hazards, infections, and other environmental factors. People with this type of asthma are likely to have a chronic or recurrent wheeze, reflecting their ongoing difficulties with breathing.

In either case, however, if you have asthma, you must learn what allergies, environmental factors, and emotional issues affect you. You must learn what you can do to build up your system, to prevent and respond to attacks. Ask not "What is asthma?" or even "What is *my* asthma?" but rather, "Who am I with asthma?"

### *Questions to Ask Your Doctor about* Your *Asthma*

- Do I have any nasal problems that are affecting my breathing—and, ultimately, my asthma?
- Are there any other factors affecting my breathing?
- Are you sure that I have asthma? How do you know? What other conditions have you ruled out? Why?
- What tests, if any, do I need to diagnose my condition? What does the test measure? Why will that be helpful?
- Have I been tested for allergies? Are allergies contributing to my asthma?

- What are my test results? Can you explain what you found and why it is significant?
- Do I have any complications that we must also address?
- Do I have any infections that we must also address?
- Do you think that I have any permanent changes? What type? How much?
- What observations of myself and my experience can I make that would be helpful to you in figuring out my diagnosis and my treatment?
- What observations can I make that you think might be helpful to *me*?

# 3

# You Can Take Action

Over the years, Paul has met lots of children with asthma. His friend Jamal has asthma, but Jamal plays soccer and seems to be able to participate in lots of games and activities that Paul is afraid to join in. Paul's cousin Miriam also has asthma, as does Miriam's friend Jason. Paul also knows grownups with asthma–his first-grade teacher, a man who works in the neighborhood candy store, and Aunt Jean, his father's sister.

Paul's mother had asthma when she was a child, but she seems to have outgrown it. She says that when she was a little girl, she was the only person she knew–child or grownup–who had asthma. She and Paul wonder whether it's just a coincidence that Paul knows so many people with asthma.

## Prevalence of Asthma Shows Striking Increase

Paul and his mother might be surprised to know that Paul's experience is no coincidence. Asthma really has become far more common than ever before.

When asthma was first identified about a century ago, it was a relatively rare disease. Then, in the 1970s, for reasons we don't fully understand, asthma began to become far more common–and far more deadly. While heart disease and cancer remain the top two causes of death in the United States, lung disease is now this country's number-three killer. Moreover, while death rates for heart disease and cancer (except lung cancer) are falling, death rates for lung disease are rising. Between 1979 and 1992, the rate of death from heart disease fell by nearly 28 percent. During the same period, the death rate from lung disease rose by 17.5 percent.

Lung disease includes pneumonia, various types of lung cancers, bronchitis, and tuberculosis, all acute and dramatic conditions generally recognized as potentially deadly. But the category of fatal lung disease also includes the chronic condition of asthma, which in 1997 caused 6,890 deaths according to the Centers for Disease Control.

Chronic bronchitis, emphysema, and asthma all obstruct the airways. Some 20 percent of U.S. citizens—40 million people—suffer from some type of obstructed airways. This number includes 15 million with asthma, 4.8 million of whom are children.

Asthma is not generally recognized as a fatal disease, yet fatalities from asthma are on the rise. The number of deaths caused by asthma has nearly doubled since 1978. In the United States, the number of hospital admissions for treatment of asthma symptoms has also shot up dramatically. From 1970 to 1980, the number of hospital visits because of asthma rose almost threefold, whereas the number of visits related to other childhood diseases remained stable. In 1992, hospitals recorded some 1.5 million asthma-related emergency room visits. Throughout the 1990s, at least 500,000 people were hospitalized with asthma each year.

Meanwhile, the incidence of asthma continues to increase, rising by more than 40 percent since 1982. According to the Bureau of Health Statistics, the rate has increased by 61 percent since the early 1980s.

In young people, the rate of increase is even more arresting: some 7 percent of all children have asthma, up 73 percent from 1982 to 1994. Even among middle-aged people, who were once relatively unusual candidates for asthma, the incidence of the disease has risen 24 percent in the last decade. Some 5 percent of all adults develop asthma—though some of these may have had asthma as children that was temporarily in remission.

### *The Poverty Connection*

The effects of asthma are even more severe in certain populations. For a variety of reasons, African Americans are disproportionately affected by asthma and are particularly susceptible to fatalities from that illness. Although they represent only 12 percent of the U.S. population, they account for some 21 percent of asthma-related deaths. And the problem is getting worse: in 1979, African Americans were about twice as likely to die from asthma as were white people; by 1987, they were three times as likely. Among people age fifteen to forty-four, the African American death rate is nearly five times higher than the white rate. In urban centers, the gap widens still more: the death rate from asthma in East Harlem, a poor African American and Latino neighborhood in New York City, is nearly ten times the national average.

The rise of asthma actually corresponds to the increasing gap between the rich and poor in the United States. According to the National Bureau of Health Statistics, between 1979 and 1988, nearly 1 million families headed by women fell below the poverty line, so that now, nearly half the families headed by women are poor. For families headed by African American women, the figure is three-quarters. During the same period, asthma was up significantly—and its rise was particularly substantial among women. In 1980, some 32 males per 1,000 had asthma, as compared to only 30 women per 1,000. By 1990, however, some 45 women per 1,000 had asthma, as opposed to only 40 men. The number of men dying of asthma rose by 23 percent in the 1980s—but during the same period, the number of women dying of asthma rose by 54 percent. Clearly, asthma and poverty are intimately related. The role of exposure to tobacco smoke is not clear, but smoking is more common in lower socioeconomic households and smoking has increased among females.

Children of all races tend to suffer from asthma at a remarkably greater rate than adults—although, as the prevalence of the disease increases, the growing numbers of adults with asthma are bringing the two rates closer together. In 1992, more than 63 children per 1,000 suffered from asthma, while nearly 45 per 1,000 adults age eighteen to forty-four suffered from the disease. In young people under age fifteen, asthma is the most common reason for hospitalization due to chronic disease, and it's the most common cause of school absences due to chronic conditions. It is the leading serious chronic illness for all U.S. children.

## The Costs of Asthma

The increasing prevalence of asthma is putting an enormous strain on our health care system. In 1985, office-based physicians recorded only 6.5 million asthma-related visits; by 1992, this figure had risen to 9.7 million. In direct health care expense alone, asthma costs our nation nearly $7 billion, including $1.6 billion in in-patient hospital care, and $1 billion in medications.

Moreover, asthma costs us $2.6 billion a year in lost productivity. Adults lost nearly 3 million workdays from asthma in 1990, while children lost 10 million school days. According to the National Center for Health Statistics, adults with asthma lose $850 million in wages each year, while parents with asthma lose $1 billion in child-care costs.

Asthma is the seventh-ranking chronic condition in the United States, besides being the leading serious chronic condition for children.

# Why Our Family? Why Now?

The most painful question that the person with asthma can ask is Why me? Why am I burdened with this frustrating disease, which at best requires me to take so much trouble over activities that other people take for granted, which at worst limits my life in painful and debilitating ways?

This is a painful question because there really are no answers. No one understands why, for example, two fraternal twins, with remarkably similar genetic material, growing up in the same environment, eating the same foods, don't both develop the same diseases. No one understands why some people are born with unusually sensitive lungs or with highly reactive immune systems, or why some of those people develop asthma while others don't.

Furthermore, no one understands why we as a society are facing this unprecedented rise in the incidence and fatality of asthma. As asthma specialist and author Dr. Richard N. Firshein puts it, "Asthma no longer plays by the rules doctors have used to describe it for the last two thousand years." In the past, most children *did* outgrow their asthma; now, in the words of Dutch researcher Dr. Ruurd Van Roorda, "When you have asthma, you always have asthma." In the past, asthma was considered a frustrating but not a particularly fatal disease. It is speculated that the increase in smoking by women has led to increased exposure of children as well as contributed to the rise in asthma in females.

## *Asthma and Industry*

Ironically, the very process of industrial development that has lengthened our life span and freed us from so many debilitating diseases seems to be intimately bound up with the dramatic rise in asthma. Nonindustrial countries seem remarkably free of asthma, which then bursts onto the scene the moment that development begins. A 1991 UNESCO study of children in Zimbabwe, for example, found that only 1 in 1,000 rural children were afflicted with asthma, whereas 1 in 17, or 5.8 percent, of the children in prosperous sections of the capital city of Harare suffered from asthma.

Likewise, in Papua New Guinea, the rate of asthma rose from virtually zero to over 7 percent in the last two decades. The increase seems to be related to recent availability of blankets, which previously had been unknown in the area. Before "development," dust mites had nowhere to nest. The blankets, however, offered the mites a haven—and the new concentration of the mites in turn triggered attacks of asthma.

Urban development is certainly associated with asthma. Only 5.5 percent of all U.S. citizens have asthma—but the rate goes up to 8.4 percent in New York City, and can be as high as 25 percent in New York's poorest neighborhoods.

It's tempting to look at air pollution as the culprit. Certainly, on bad-air days, hospitals report more asthma-related admissions—as many as 20 to 30 percent more than when air is "normal." But in industrial nations, air pollution has been vastly reduced over the past century—think of the blinding "pea-soup" fogs in nineteenth-century London, caused by the dust and fumes in the air—which should have helped asthma rates to go down, not up. Even as late as the 1950s, Londoners suffered from increased rates of bronchitis because of their city's polluted air. Bronchitis rates fell as the air got cleaner—but asthma rates shot up. Likewise, East German children have a lower rate of asthma than their counterparts in West Germany, even though they are exposed to up to ten times more air pollution. Again, the role of tobacco smoking may have prevented the expected drop related to air pollution.

The underlying causes of asthma appear to be related to industrial development in more subtle and far-reaching ways. Think of the three signs of "gracious living" that became common in developed nations after World War II: central heating, wall-to-wall carpeting, and double-glazed windows. The heating and insulation keep air inside the house, rather than letting it circulate and purge itself of pollutants. And, thanks to the wonders of modern science, indoor air is more polluted than ever before. That wall-to-wall carpeting collects dust, providing a breeding ground for the dust mites that trigger asthma. Meanwhile, we clean our bathrooms and kitchens with industrial-strength cleansers; dry-clean our clothes with chemicals; air-condition and dehumidify our homes with mold-breeding appliances; and, unlike previous generations, bring our cats and dogs inside the house to live with us. On the one hand, we've exponentially increased the number of asthma triggers inside our homes (and offices); on the other hand, we've done a fabulous job of sealing those pollutants—including tobacco smoke—inside the house with us.

### *The Indoor Life*

At the same time, our children stay indoors to a far greater extent, vastly increasing their exposure to allergens and irritants. In the 1960s, American children played outdoors for an average of three hours a day; now, thanks to video games, television, and other home entertainments, the average is only two hours. Sedentary, indoor children grow up to be the same kind of adult: according to the Environmental Protection Agency, most U.S. adults spend 90 percent of their time indoors—and the rest of their time in cars.

Because more adults are working full-time, more children are in day care and preschool—and at earlier ages than ever before. About one-third of U.S. three- and four-year-olds are in some kind of group care, and the figure is even higher elsewhere in the industrialized world. The greater concentration of children means that the children tend to "share" their illnesses as well as their toys—and some scientists believe that a higher rate of infection with certain respiratory viruses makes a child more likely to contract asthma. On the other hand, one study suggested that early infections actually led to a decrease in asthma later on.

## *Asthma and Additives*

Some asthma experts believe that nutrition is also a key issue. They point out that with the rise of development, both children and adults eat far less fresh fruit and vegetables, and far more additives and preservatives. Children may be deprived of essential nutrients early in life. Adults, too, may be reacting to this nutritional imbalance, with the result that both children and adults are far more susceptible to asthma.

## *The Role of Modern Medicine*

Ironically, modern medicine itself may have made the problem worse. By masking the symptoms of asthma, over-the-counter inhalers allowed many people with asthma to get sicker and sicker. As long as people with asthma could use inhalers to help them breathe, they could ignore the fact that their lungs were becoming more and more inflamed—to the point that someday an inhaler would not help. One Canadian study found that people with asthma who inhaled thirteen or more canisters in a year—about one per month—increased their risk of dying ninetyfold. True, thirteen canisters a year is higher than the recommended dose—but many people with asthma, wanting the relief that an inhaler offers, do exceed the recommended dose to that extent.

By teaching their patients to rely on the wonders of modern pharmacology, many doctors were actually encouraging them to remain in the environments or homes that were making them sick, to continue the lifestyle choices that were supporting the disease. Many doctors simply prescribed medication, unsupported by breathing exercises, changes in diet, healthy exercise regimes, and the like—often at the behest of patients who were delighted to find such "simple" cures. Imagine treating a diabetic by prescribing ever-higher doses of insulin, while the diabetic goes on eating sweet desserts and drinking large quantities of alcohol. Or imagine treating a heart patient by prescribing the latest medications while encouraging the person to continue smoking and to eat fried foods. That, in effect, was the equivalent of how many doctors and patients approached the treatment of asthma—with predictably poor results.

## Families Coping with Asthma

In the words of Dr. Gregory Owens of the University of Pittsburgh School of Medicine, "Asthma is perhaps one of the most underrated and undertreated of all the major diseases that afflict human beings." For a person suffering with asthma—or for a parent whose child is suffering—it can be frustrating to try to understand and treat the disease.

Frequently, asthma is not diagnosed properly—or not diagnosed at all. It is relatively difficult to diagnose in children. Many childhood diseases mimic asthma. Other conditions, such as gastroesophageal reflux, may aggravate asthma symptoms. Sometimes a pediatrician fears telling parents that their child has asthma, because of the "overprotective" or panicked reaction that he or she imagines that parents will have. In other cases, doctors make a point of diagnosing a childhood condition as asthma in order to shock parents into, say, giving up smoking or making other radical changes to benefit the child. Children with mild symptoms of asthma such as chest pain or discomfort after exercising may simply cope with the symptoms on their own—say, by avoiding exercise—rather than telling an adult about the problem.

Asthma may also be difficult to diagnose in adults. Many doctors aren't aware of the recent rise in adult-onset asthma. They may not realize that frequent chest infections or bouts of bronchitis or persistent cough often indicate asthma.

## Understanding Asthma

Even when asthma is properly diagnosed, it is often not understood, either by doctors or by lay people. Many people believe that asthma is "all psychological" or that it's primarily caused by overprotective parents. People who would never dream of insisting that a person with diabetes eat dessert feel comfortable insisting that a person with asthma stay in a room where a dog or cat has been. Smokers often don't realize that secondary cigarette smoke can indeed be deadly for people with asthma–particularly for children who have asthma. They don't realize that smoke lingers in the air, so that the cigarette they had that morning may bring on an asthma attack in the evening.

People with asthma often feel ambivalent about their condition. On the one hand, if you have asthma, you know you're suffering. On the other hand, you, too, may think that it's "all in your mind," a sign of how badly you handle stress, an indication of how overly sensitive or fussy you are. You may simply get tired of asking friends not to smoke, of making detailed inquiries about pets and houseplants, of interrogating waiters about potential allergens lurking in your restaurant meal. You may feel that the annoyance or oversolicitousness of your loved ones is wearing or intrusive or simply upsetting.

## Parents and Asthma

Parents of children with asthma are likely to have a whole host of contradictory, disturbing feelings. First, of course, there's the gut-level concern for your child, whom you are responsible for protecting. Then there's the self-doubt: Should you be doing more? Should you be doing less? Are you being overprotective? Underprotective? Have you missed some obvious treatment that might help? Some obvious trigger that, once removed, will make life better for your child? If you have other children, you probably wonder whether you are slighting them in favor of the child with asthma, who may be more needy, or who may feel more needy.

### *A Holistic Approach*

Dealing with your reactions to asthma—and with other people's reactions to it—is a central part of coping with the disease. You are not just a collection of symptoms; you are a whole person, living a full life, within which asthma affects your relationships and your feelings as well as your throat and your lungs. If you're a parent of a child with asthma, one of the best things you can do for your child is to understand your own contradictory feelings while helping your child sort through his or her mixed emotions. (For more about asthma and emotion, see Chapter 8. For more about children with asthma, see Chapter 13.)

## "What Can I Do?"

Any effective approach to treating asthma will have three components:

1. Understand the disease.
2. Understand yourself.
3. Take action.

### *Understand the Disease*

The more you know about how asthma works, what sets it off, and what might ease its effects, the more effectively you can respond to it. Obviously, knowing about your condition can help you make informed decisions about what kind of treatment you need and what steps you might take to prevent an attack. But beyond the specific facts, knowledge brings a more general benefit: responsibility. People who understand their condition have taken the first step on the road to responsible self-care, toward beginning to heal themselves. It may be tempting to sit back, relax, and let a doctor make all of your health care decisions, but the process is not nearly as healing as one in which you take an active responsibility for your own health.

## *Understand Yourself*

It's not helpful to understand any "disease" as some external force that has to be fought off. It's far more effective to see any physical condition—whether health or sickness—as an aspect of yourself.

Let's be very clear: You have not caused your asthma, you have not somehow willed it or brought it on yourself because of a faulty personality or some kind of "wish" to be sick. Being sick is an experience like any other. The more you understand this experience and make it your own, the more you can shape the experience in the direction that you choose. In other words, understanding yourself as someone with asthma is more helpful than simply understanding "asthma" as some outside force.

What does this mean in practice? It means knowing your body and knowing what affects you. Perhaps you wake up one morning feeling unusually sensitive; that may be a day to avoid a busy, polluted street that, on a less sensitive day, would not bother you at all. Perhaps you are especially affected by lack of sleep, so on short-sleep days, you pay special attention to diet and food allergies. One of the most frightening aspects of asthma is its abruptness: people are often unexpectedly overcome by an attack or are surprised by a violent reaction to a particular food or odor. You may not be able to entirely prevent those experiences—but you may be able to know far more about them than you realize.

Tim Brookes, author of a personal account of asthma, *Catching My Breath*, attributes his ability to achieve a virtually asthma-free life to his exploration of the disease and his own relationship to it. He believes that by writing about his condition, he was able to transform it. Self-knowledge became the route to self-healing. Brookes, who calls himself a "recovering asthmatic," comments on what he sees as the value of the few asthmatic symptoms that he still experiences: "This remnant of asthma is a form of perception: it amplifies, in a sense, emotions that I might be disposed to ignore or suppress." Asthma, he feels, helps to draw his attention inward, so that he can hear sounds "that are beyond the audible range."

Brookes also gives full credit to the inhaled steroids he began to take after a near-fatal asthma attack. He points out that he never strays too far from his inhaler, and that he'll never live too far from an emergency room. But, he writes, people with asthma might find strength and healing power in thinking of illness as an activity—an activity to be undertaken with curiosity. Brookes likens being an "active patient" to being someone who fixes his or her own car: a person who greets odd sounds and the occasional breakdown as a chance to find out more, to tinker and experiment, to learn more about the early warning signs of trouble. In his own experience, this attitude helped him to become "less fearful of life and death" as well as more patient with himself, "more respectful of being ill."

After all, Brookes points out, everyone's health is only temporary. All of us, whether we have asthma or not, live on the razor's edge between health and sickness. All of us, no matter what our physical condition, can benefit from getting to know our bodies, through both study and experience, as well as getting to know what physical and emotional conditions affect our state of health and our state of mind.

An enormous body of information about asthma exists "out there": reports of doctors' experiences and scientists' studies. But you also have within you an enormous "body of information" about *your* asthma, about *you*, as a body that happens to include asthma. Just the process of getting to know your own individual experience will help you to "breathe easier," in both senses of the word. And, of course, the more you know, the better choices you can make.

### *Take Action*

What choices can you make to lessen your asthma and prevent attacks? You'll find out more in subsequent chapters that discuss allergens to avoid (Chapter 4), environmental factors to clean up or avoid (Chapters 6 and 7), healthy lifestyle choices (Chapters 8 and 9), effective ways to use medication (Chapter 11), and alternative treatments to explore (Chapter 12). Here, however, is a brief overview of action that you can take:

- *Clean up your environment at home.* Find out what allergens are attacking you where you live—and learn how you can eliminate or restrict them.
- *Clean up your environment at work.* If exposures at work are making you sick, what can you do about it? Your options may include switching offices, wearing a protective mask, or altering your environment in some way. It's also possible that diet, exercise, or reducing exposure at home may make you less sensitive to work-related exacerbants.
- *Improve your diet.* Certain vitamin and mineral supplements seem to help increase the body's resistance to asthma triggers. And a low-fat diet, rich in complex carbohydrates and a wide variety of vegetables, can contribute to overall health.
- *Develop a healthy exercise pattern.* Exercising your lungs, as well as your heart and your other muscles, can help combat asthma in all sorts of ways. A few simple precautions can help you avoid exercise-induced asthma as you create the exercise routine that is right for you.
- *Learn how to breathe properly.* Amazingly, many people with asthma have never consciously worked on their breathing. Although faulty breathing in no way causes asthma or triggers an attack, proper breathing can help prevent attacks as well as lessen their effects.

## Working with Your Doctor

Clearly, the approach to healing and self-care outlined here depends on developing a proactive, responsible relationship with your physician. Such a relationship, in turn, must be based on mutual trust and respect.

All too often, the doctor-patient relationship has been founded on an all-powerful doctor and a submissive patient, in which the doctor's role is to give orders and the patient's role is to follow them. Patients often have mixed feelings about this relationship: on the one hand, they may feel safe and secure in the care of the all-powerful doctor, whom they can assume knows what is best for them; on the other hand, they may feel resentful and frustrated that their own opinions are not listened to, that they don't receive adequate explanations of their condition or their treatment, or that they are being assigned a treatment that for some reason doesn't fit their lives.

As a result, patients frequently don't follow a doctor's orders. They might discontinue a course of medication as soon as they feel better, even though the doctor has explained that all the pills in a prescription must be taken. They might self-medicate, using leftover pills from an earlier prescription or even from another person's prescription. They might take fewer pills than the doctor has prescribed, or take pills more often or under different conditions than they've been told. They might ignore a doctor's recommendation for diet, exercise, and lifestyle changes—and they might even lie to the doctor about their behavior in order to seem like "good patients."

On the other hand, although many doctors are dedicated, sensitive, and respectful of their patients, some are not. Doctors may forget that although they have seen several hundred asthma patients, to any individual patient, the information is new and the experience of illness is all too personal. Doctors may also focus exclusively on information and action, forgetting that for virtually everyone with asthma, the disease is an overwhelmingly emotional experience.

What's the solution? Envision the kind of relationship you'd like with your physician, and then work actively to develop such a relationship. Perhaps you can create a good relationship with the doctor you're already seeing; if this isn't possible, you may need to look for a new doctor. Here are the responsibilities inherent in each side of the doctor-patient relationship:

**Doctors should:**

- Fully explain what they know about the patient's condition.
- Be honest about what they don't know.
- Involve the patient to the fullest extent possible in making choices regarding treatment, based on sharing information with the patient about medication and lifestyle changes.
- Be willing to explore diet, exercise, lifestyle changes, and alternative treatments as possible supplements to medication, with the goal of eventually reducing medication as far as possible.
- Be sensitive to the patient's emotional experience of asthma.
- Be clear, specific, and flexible about the patient's treatment.

**Patients should:**

- Be willing to learn about their condition, both through study and through paying attention to their own experiences.
- Keep careful records of their own experiences, both for their own information and to share information and insights with the doctor.
- Be willing to work with a physician who also has questions and uncertainties.
- Take an active role in considering and choosing treatments.
- Be honest about what they have and have not done, with regard to taking medications, making lifestyle changes, and the like.
- Be honest about what they are and are not willing to do, with regard to following a doctor's suggestions or agreeing to a treatment plan.
- Be willing to ask questions, express their feelings, and continue a discussion until both they and the doctor are satisfied with the outcome.

### *Keep an Asthma Journal*

One of the best ways to get to know your condition—and to gather information of use to your physician—is to keep an asthma journal. Each day for two weeks, at the end of the day, take note of how you felt. Include information about your mood and your general outlook, and note any symptoms of asthma, allergies, or infections. Note what you ate, what the weather was, where you were, and what activities you engaged in. Be as specific as possible: noting when you experienced an asthma symptom (right after that upsetting phone call with your boss? two hours after that Chinese meal?) might help you or your doctor figure out what triggered it. You can also keep an asthma journal for your child or loved one.

### *Take an Asthma Survey*

The following survey will also help you evaluate the various aspects of your life that might be contributing to your asthma. Take the survey, and then share the results with your doctor. The two of you might be surprised at what you learn!

**Asthma Survey**

*Home*

1. In general, do you feel better at home or away from home?
2. Which rooms in your house are carpeted?
3. Do you notice symptoms in your bedroom?
4. Do you use an impermeable mattress cover? Do your pillows contain natural feathers or down?
5. Do you have forced-air central heating?
6. Do you have an air conditioner? A humidifier or dehumidifier?
7. Do you notice symptoms in your bathroom?
8. Which, if any, of the following substances seem to produce asthma symptoms? Soaps, solvents, bleaches, ammonia, polishes, floor waxes, moth balls, varnish, hair

## You Can Take Action

spray, perfumes (including the ones in magazine strips), newsprint?

9. Does anyone in your family have a hobby that involves using glue, paint, cleaners, or solvents?
10. Do you feel worse after using the vacuum cleaner?
11. Was your home recently renovated? Have you installed new carpet, painted, or bought new furniture?

*Workplace*

1. In general, do you feel better or worse at work?
2. Do you work near a photocopy machine or laser printer?
3. Do you work with paints, solvents, cleaners, inks, dyes, or glues?
4. Does anyone in your workplace smoke?
5. Is your workplace well ventilated?
6. Is the ventilation system buildingwide?
7. Is your workplace heated by forced air?
8. Is your workplace air-conditioned?

*Food*

1. Do you crave any particular foods or sweets? Which are they?
2. Are you currently taking vitamins, minerals, or herbal supplements? Which are they? What brands are they? What dosages do you take? Check the labels: what fillers or ingredients do they include?
3. Do you drink alcohol? More than twice a week?
4. How many servings of fresh vegetables do you eat each day? How many servings of fruit?
5. How often do you eat junk food? What kind do you eat? What time of day do you eat it?
6. Which, if any, of the following symptoms do you notice immediately after eating? Fatigue, shortness of breath,

wheezing, stuffy nose, runny nose, hives, itching, flushing, feeling hot, feeling cold?

***Allergies***

1. Have you ever tested positive on allergy tests? Were they prick, scratch, or blood tests?
2. Have you been tested for allergens within the past year? Which allergens, molds, foods, pollens, and other substances did you test positive for?
3. Are you currently being treated for allergies? How?
4. Do you notice allergy symptoms at certain times of day or times of year?
5. Do you react with symptoms to animals?
6. Do you suffer from cluster headaches or migraines?
7. Are you bothered by damp rooms? By damp days?
8. Do you live near a wooded area or open field?

***Ask Your Doctor . . .***

Because the doctor-patient relationship is so important, every subsequent chapter in this book ends with a set of questions that you can use to open up a conversation with your physician. To find out your doctor's general approach to asthma, and to discover the kind of doctor-patient relationship the two of you might have, the following questions might be helpful:

- What's your prognosis for the extent to which I can live an active, "normal" life?
- What, if any, limits in my life do you think I have to be prepared to accept?
- What's your goal for my use of medication? If this treatment goes as you hope, what medication will I use, how much, and how often?
- What is your view of the relationship between diet, exercise, lifestyle choices, and asthma?

- What is your view on alternative approaches, such as meditation, biofeedback, chiropractic, acupuncture, and hypnosis?
- I'm interested in keeping an asthma journal in order to find out more about how, when, and why I react to various asthma triggers. How should I share the information from that journal with you?
- What kind of doctor-patient relationship would you like us to have? What do you think your responsibilities are toward me? What do you think my responsibilities are toward you?
- What kinds of environments, foods, or other triggers are setting off my asthma attacks?
- What kinds of action do you think I can take to reduce the number of asthma triggers in my environment?
- What can I do to learn more about asthma?

# 4

# Understanding the Allergy-Asthma Connection

Malcolm always considered that his allergies made up a very short list, a short list that he could control. He knew exactly what he had to avoid as far as foods were concerned: peanuts and shrimp. And as long as he stayed away from cats and dogs, he was just fine.

Then Malcolm got a promotion at work, and was moved to a newly renovated corner office. Suddenly, he was coughing and sneezing all the time—and sometimes, the coughing turned into an asthma attack. Malcolm is sure that no pets have ever been in his office. But clearly, he is having an allergic—and occasionally an asthmatic—reaction to that space.

About two weeks after moving into the new office, Malcolm noticed that he often wakes up stuffy and congested. A few weeks after that, he begins waking up in the middle of the night, coughing, sneezing, and unable to catch his breath. Sometimes these nighttime interruptions turn into full-blown asthma attacks. Other times, they hover just on the edge of an attack, but they do interfere with Malcolm's sleep—and with his peace of mind.

The last straw is that lately, Malcolm has been having allergic—and sometimes asthmatic—reactions to restaurant meals. He frequently takes clients out to lunch or dinner, and he likes to let them choose the restaurant. Malcolm's first reaction occurred after a meal at a Chinese restaurant, so he thought that maybe he was just having a reaction to MSG. Then he had a strong reaction at a Thai restaurant, even though he was careful not to order anything with peanuts in it. Having lunch one day at a "standard American" luxury restaurant, Malcolm ordered some homemade wild mushroom soup—and began coughing and sneezing as soon as he took the first taste. He just doesn't understand why all of a sudden, he is having so many allergic reactions.

## Allergens, Atopy, and Asthma

Malcolm is not alone. Some 50 percent of people with asthma over age thirty are strongly allergic. Younger people with asthma are even more likely to be allergic: 70 percent of those under age thirty and 90 percent of those under sixteen have allergies. People with asthma may be allergic to dust mites, cockroaches, animals, plants, pollen, molds, chemicals, or additives. Wood smoke and cigarette smoke may contribute by irritating airways.

Both asthma and allergic reactions tend to run in families. Indeed, the condition known as *atopy* (from the Greek meaning uncommon or changed reaction) includes a tendency to hay fever, skin rash, asthma, and allergies, seems to appear along familial lines. And in families where parents, especially mothers, have either asthma or atopy, the children are more likely to have either one or both conditions. Although we don't know exactly how this works, asthma seems to have some connection with the allergic reactions of hay fever and eczema, as well as with pneumonia, bronchitis, and migraine. Many children who have hay fever or eczema eventually develop asthma.

Some people with asthma never suffer from allergies. Other people may have frequent asthmatic reactions whenever they come in contact with a food or substance to which they're allergic. Still other people have allergic reactions involving the nose or skin that turn into asthmatic reactions at other times.

### *New Allergies*

As Malcolm is discovering, people may suddenly develop allergies to substances that never used to bother them. Allergies may spontaneously improve, but they more often spontaneously get worse. In part, that's because as a person's system becomes hyperresponsive, it becomes more and *more* hyperresponsive. As the immune system jumps quickly to what it perceives as the body's defense, it tends to jump ever more quickly. As Malcolm found, initially only animal dander is perceived as a threat; later, perhaps it's down pillows or the dust that collects in wool blankets. One day, Malcolm would have an allergic reaction only if he actually ate a peanut; later, he might have an allergic reaction to eating food cooked in the same pan where peanuts once were (which is possibly what happened at the Thai restaurant).

## *Allergies and the Downward Spiral*

Looking at Malcolm's story, we can speculate about the kind of downward spiral that his allergies have created. His renovated office probably contained allergens in the air ducts and chemical fumes that his old office didn't have. The office is newly carpeted, for example, and carpets give off fumes and collect dust. Perhaps there are some lingering paint fumes there as well. (For more about environmental factors in asthma, see Chapters 6 and 7.) These new environmental factors may have been enough to put Malcolm's system on overload. Suddenly, he is reacting violently to things that never used to bother him before, such as the down pillows in his bedroom or the traces of peanut oil left in the frying pan where his peanut-free noodles were sauteed.

Thus, by the time he had lunch at the "standard American" restaurant, Malcolm's system had already been "insulted" several times by potent allergens/asthma triggers. Malcolm was told that the restaurant's mushroom soup was freshly made, but the soup actually contained canned chicken stock, which included sulfites, an additive that sets off strong reactions in many people with asthma. Malcolm had eaten foods with sulfites before with no ill consequences. Now, though, weakened both by repeated exposure to other allergens as well as by lack of sleep (from those other late-night asthma attacks), Malcolm's system is more sensitive, quicker to react, and so the sulfites set off a powerful physical reaction.

## Physical and Emotional Reactions

At a certain point, the physical reaction becomes an emotional one. Malcolm is starting to feel that he can't do anything without running the risk of an asthma attack. For someone so proud of not letting his asthma control him, this is doubly bitter knowledge. Not only does Malcolm have to fear unexpected asthma attacks or, at the very least, bouts of coughing, choking, and congestion, he also has to struggle with his own feelings of failure that he really can't control his condition.

# "Do I Have Allergies?"

One of the most insidious things about allergies is the way they soon come to seem "normal." We grow used to a certain level of discomfort, ill-health, and reduced vitality, particularly when we don't know what's causing the problem or when we don't take the cause seriously. For some reason, people who would respect a diabetic's strong reaction to sugar or an alcoholic's problematic relationship to liquor often pooh-pooh an allergic person's equally violent responses to allergens. We tend to think that people with allergies are simply being "difficult," "overly sensitive," or "fussy"–and if we ourselves have allergies, we may be even less forgiving.

At the same time, we may not even realize the myriad ways that allergies can sap our energy and lower our sense of bodily ease. Here are some of the many parts of the body that are affected by various allergies:

- *Nose.* Rhinitis set off by allergies can lead to an itchy, runny, or stopped-up nose and mucus may drain into the back of the throat.
- *Sinuses.* Sinusitis can lead to the feeling that your whole head is congested. In some cases, it also causes headache. Sinusitis produces mucus, which, if it drips down into the throat, can bring on a fit of coughing, interfere with sleep, and in some cases, trigger an asthma attack.

- *Eyes.* Conjunctivitis can cause the eyes to itch, tear, or turn red.
- *Skin.* A condition known as urticaria or hives causes itching and swelling as one type of allergic reaction.
- *Stomach and intestines.* Allergic reactions to food and other substances can lead to gastroenteritis, which includes nausea, cramping, and diarrhea.
- *Bloodstream.* The most severe type of allergic reaction, anaphylaxis, includes falling blood pressure, sweating, and other total-body symptoms. A person who goes into anaphylactic shock, in which blood pressure falls extremely rapidly, might die within a few minutes if not properly treated.
- *Laryngeal area.* Swelling can close off the upper airway, causing a stridor, or high-pitched noise, during inspiration and expiration.
- *Lungs.* Allergic disturbances felt in the lungs including wheezing, coughing, excess production of mucus, and, of course, asthma itself.

Do any of these symptoms sound familiar to you? Have you grown used to indigestion or sore eyes, never thinking that you might be having an allergic reaction? You might explore whether you have allergies, particularly if there is a history of allergy in your family or if there is any seasonal pattern to your allergies. Winter tends to be the most allergy-free season for pollen-sensitive people, although we usually spend long periods of time indoors; the air that circulates continuously throughout the house, retaining dust mites, mold, and chemical fumes from carpets, dry cleaning, and household products, causes particular problems for dust mite-sensitive people. In spring, the trees produce pollen–and allergens. In the summer, grass pollen sets off some people's allergies. Fall often brings a harvest of weeds that in turn bring on hay fever and other allergic reactions. Even if you feel symptom-free at the moment, look back over the list you just read and consider whether you might have been sustaining a load of allergies all these years, without even realizing it.

## Allergies, Your Immune System, and Asthma

What exactly happens when an allergen invades your system? As with many other key questions, scientists are still trying to figure out more about this complicated and lengthy process. Here is the current theory of what happens:

Allergens that may be inhaled, eaten, or touched enter the body and encounter enzymes or chemicals in mucus or saliva that may break down the proteins into smaller components that are then absorbed into the circulation or into the lymphatic system. In the subcutaneous tissues or the tissues in airways or intestines are mast cells, which are critical to the allergic and asthmatic reaction. If the person is genetically programmed to produce immunoglobulin E (IgE) antibodies, these are attached to the mast cells. If these antibodies are directed against the allergen, this process leads to release of mediators, or chemicals that have potent effects.

There's a lot we don't know about this stage of the immune process. For example, some antibodies, such as IgE, seem to do the body more harm than good. One theory is that they were developed by the body to fight against parasites and perhaps other invaders that no longer exist in nature, so that the body is equipped with "weapons systems" that don't match current enemies. Absent their proper targets, these antibodies instead signal a chemical reaction that attacks the body.

We do know that DNA–genetic programming–is what directs the B-cells to make various types of antibodies. In a properly functioning body, once enough IgM is made, the B-cells are supposed to switch to IgG. Only 1 percent of their output is supposed to be IgE. In some people, however, the DNA programming seems to be mixed up. These people may make from ten to twenty times more IgE than other people make. These may be people who have overly sensitive immune systems—which translates into allergies and asthma.

1. The specific IgE attaches to *mast cells,* the "gatekeepers" of the body. The greatest concentration of mast cells is found just under the skin, and in the nasal passages, lungs, and intestines. In other words, if you are scratched, breathe in poison, or eat something that's bad for you, the mast cells will be right there in the area, ready to react. (At least, they will be ready once they have been signaled by the specific IgE or by some nonspecific types such as opiate drugs.)

2. So the tiny IgE antibody feels its way around, say, the lung's epithelium—the delicate skin that lines the airways. It finds a mast cell to which it can attach itself. This process of attachment alerts the mast cell, which is studded with tiny granules, each containing powerful chemicals. These chemicals' job is either to fight infection, or to tell some other chemical to do so. Scientists call this the *inflammatory cascade,* because each chemical seems to call forth another, in a cascade of chemical reactions that produces inflammation.

3. One mast cell chemical, for example, is *histamine.* (If you've suffered from colds or allergic reactions, you may have taken an *antihistamine.*) Histamine makes the small blood vessels expand, so that the cells don't fit together snugly. Fluid and lymphocytes are thus free to slide out of the blood into the surrounding tissue, where they can hunt for invaders. The downside is that the increase of fluid in the tissue also causes swelling. And when this swelling occurs in the epithelium, it narrows the airways—which makes breathing difficult.

4. The lungs react to swelling by producing more mucus. What they intended to do was smooth the passage of air into and out of the lungs. What they accomplished was to clog themselves with mucus, making breathing even more difficult than before.

5. Histamine has another side effect: it causes the smooth muscles around the bronchial tube to contract. This bronchoconstriction narrows the airways still further. Now, breathing is even more difficult.

Allergies, then, result from the interaction of IgE antibodies and mast cells. An allergic person's body contains IgE antibodies that are sensitized to hundreds, maybe thousands, of substances—cat dander, mold, pollen, dust mites, wood smoke—the list goes on and on. And, as Malcolm is learning, the list can get longer at any time. As someone whose body has produced lots of extra IgE, Malcolm has B cells that are just waiting to be sensitized to various "invaders" and to produce specific IgE antibodies.

Scientists don't exactly know why some people are so overly sensitized to their environments. Some see people with allergies and/or asthma as "the canary in the coal mine": the people who are sensitive to substances in our environment that other people absorb without reaction.

Other scientists speculate that people with allergies and/or asthma have extra mast cells. Still others believe that some people's mast cells have migrated to the surface of their lungs, causing particular trouble with airborne allergens.

Clearly, this is a realm of science that is marked by more questions than answers. But we do know just a bit more about how IgE and mast cells combine to produce an allergic/asthmatic reaction.

6. Let's take a step backward. Let's recall the very first time that a person with allergies and/or asthma inhaled, say, the waste product of a dust mite. This microscopic pellet set off an immune-system reaction culminating in thousands of tiny IgE antibodies attaching themselves to mast cells in the lungs. What happens the next time that one—or a hundred, or a hundred thousand—dust mite pellets are inhaled? Most people do inhale dust, which contains the pellets, every day. But asthmatics, with their extra IgE, have "instructed" their mast cells to react to pellets. In other words, the IgE attached to the mast cell detects the dust mite pellet and "tells" the mast cell to do its job. Immediately, mast cells release the inflammatory cascade, a whole host of chemicals, histamine included, that cause swelling, mucus production, smooth muscle contraction, and, eventually, the nar-

rowing of the airways that causes coughing, wheezing, and shortness of breath.

Scientists are still cataloguing all the elements involved in this inflammatory cascade. They include prostaglandins (also involved in migraines), leukotrienes, neutrophils, eosinophils, platelet-activating factors, and others, many of which are released hours or even days later. Thus inflammation of the lungs is prolonged. Even when the dust mite that started the problem has vanished completely from the lungs, the process that was set in motion may still continue.

Of course, this does not explain why allergic reactions are specific to one tissue. Why, for example, does hay fever affect the nose and not the lungs? Why does asthma affect the lungs and not the skin? And why do people have asthmatic reactions to cold weather, laughing, or exercise, as well as to dust mites, cat dander, or cigarette smoke?

These are questions with which allergists and immunologists wrestle every day. Let's leave them to it and return to the final step in the immune system's process.

7. Even after the suppressor T-cells have done their work, however, memory T- and B-cells remain in the bloodstream and lymph system. Their job is to remember the foreign invader and help mobilize the body to attack it should it ever return.

## Allergies and Infections

Remember Angela, who developed asthma after a series of infections? It seems that there may be a close relationship among asthma, allergies, and viral infections. Other organisms, such as mycoplana and chlamydia, can also cause asthma to begin. The body's attempt to fight off these organisms—the immune reaction we just explored—may also make the body more sensitive to allergens.

In other words, while fighting off her other infections, Angela's respiratory tract was more sensitive. As she walked home on the day of her first asthma attack, her reaction may have been triggered by the exhaust of the passing bus.

In general, allergies and infection are closely related. If the lining of the nose is often inflamed, for example, as the result of an allergic reaction, the sinuses are also affected as well as the lower airways. So another version of Angela's story might be that she had already developed the allergies that caused first her winter of problems and then her asthmatic reaction.

*Infections and Children* The relationship between allergies, asthma, and infection is particularly dangerous to young children. Asthma may sometimes be triggered by the respiratory syncytial virus (RSV), which causes a wide range of respiratory infections. Children with this genetic tendency to asthma frequently have wheezing and sometimes severe respiratory distress. In general, the younger the child with RSV, the more severe the reaction. Some of these children respond with elevated IgE and chronic asthma.

## Responses to Food Allergies

When discussing food, it might be more helpful to talk about "adverse reactions" rather than allergies. That's because the term allergy is somewhat controversial in scientific and medical circles. Rather than rehearse that debate here, let's discuss the three major types of adverse reactions to food:

*Anaphylactic Reaction* This can occur instantly, in response to as little as a single bite of a particular substance, and it can be deadly. Symptoms may include swelling of the lips, tongue, and throat; dizziness; difficulty breathing; vomiting and/or diarrhea. You may also have an asthma attack.

Usually, these reactions are provoked by peanuts, nuts, shellfish, eggs, or seeds. Unfortunately, although people who suffer from this type of reaction may avoid their own personal "danger foods," they may find themselves eating one by mistake. One tragic story, for example, concerned a young woman who ordered chili at a diner and died twenty minutes later, not realizing that the restaurant's chili recipe included peanut butter.

Therefore, if you are prone to such a reaction, you need to recognize the early symptoms, such as tingling on the tongue and lips. The most effective treatment is a dose of the hormone epinephrine, which you can inject yourself from a device known as an EpiPen or AnaKit. An antihistamine, such as Benadryl, may also be helpful. In fact, if you think you might suffer such a reaction, you should discuss precautions with your doctor immediately, and always have an EpiPen handy. In the event of an anaphylactic reaction, going to an emergency room might involve too long a delay. However, even if you have medicated yourself, you should always visit an emergency room after such an experience, because you might suffer a relapse.

*Allergic Reactions* These are not as strong as anaphylactic reactions, although there is some overlap between a mild anaphylactic reaction and a severe allergic response. Again, in these reactions, the lips generally swell and the bronchial tubes tighten. These reactions usually involve an overproduction of IgE, the antibody that sensitizes the mast cells to various substances. Sesame is a common trigger for such reactions. A person who is extremely sensitive might have an allergic reaction to, say, a hamburger that was fried in the same pan that had earlier been used to sauté fish in sesame oil.

*Delayed Allergic Reactions* These may either follow an immediate allergic reaction or occasionally occur in isolation six to twelve hours following an exposure.

These delayed reactions are naturally harder to detect, particularly in children, who might have eaten the "danger food" at school or at a friend's house. Sometimes, too, you might have a delayed reaction to a food during pollen season, when your allergy load is high and you already have lots of inflammatory chemicals in your bloodstream; whereas, you might eat the same food in the middle of winter and have no adverse reaction at all. The symptoms of delayed allergic reactions include skin rashes, asthma, stuffy nose, headache, irritability, nervousness, listlessness, and fatigue.

*Allergies and Cravings*

Often, it turns out that the very foods we crave are the ones to which we have an allergic reaction. If you suspect that you may be allergic to one of your favorite foods—a very difficult perception to face up to!—you might bite the bullet and do without that food for a week. You may find that both your craving and your allergic symptoms disappear. On the other hand, some patients "dislike" foods to which they are allergic. Parents frequently "push" milk because it contains calcium, but some of the children who dislike milk are having undetected allergic reactions.

## "Am I Allergic?"

If this description of allergic reactions has you wondering about yourself or a loved one, take a look at the following list of allergy symptoms. Do they seem familiar? They may be responses to allergies.

### Allergy Symptoms

- Recurrent ear, nose, and throat symptoms
- Frequent headaches between or behind the eyes
- Fatigue
- Asthma, shortness of breath
- Rash
- Earache
- Swelling, joint pain
- Frequent digestive problems: bloating, gas, diarrhea, constipation
- Aches and pains

- Itching after eating
- Frequent sore throat
- Dark circles under eyes

### *Responding to Allergies*

Once you become aware of your allergies, you can do a great deal to soothe, slow down, and in some cases, completely eliminate your allergic reactions. You can also work to keep your allergic reactions from triggering asthmatic reactions. For more on how to cope with allergies and mitigate their effects, go on to the next chapter.

### *Ask Your Doctor...*

- Do I need to be evaluated for allergies?
- Are you concerned about a pattern of infections in my history?
- Do you see any relationship between infections I've had and allergies that I have (or that you suspect I have)?
- What can I do to address the infections that seem to be making my allergies worse?
- How severe are my allergies?
- What do I seem to be allergic to?
- How can I find out more about my allergies?
- What, if any, medications should I be taking to address my allergies?
- Would allergy shots be useful to dampen my allergic responses?

# 5

# Coping with Your Allergies

Malcolm realizes that he has to learn more about what he is allergic to and how his allergies are affecting him. He starts by working with his doctor, who conducts a series of allergy tests and who also asks Malcolm to keep a complete diary of everything he eats and drinks for a short period of time.

Malcolm's doctor helps him to pinpoint many of the allergies that may have been triggered by environmental changes. But he also suspects that Malcolm has developed a number of allergies to food.

Malcolm is both frustrated and frightened: Will he ever be able to eat without fear of triggering a new allergic/asthmatic attack? Malcolm's doctor, however, is optimistic. He suggests that Malcolm start working with a nutritionist, who can help him learn more about how food affects not only his asthma but also his entire sense of well-being.

## Allergies and Awareness

Allergies and asthma are both highly dynamic processes, not simple chains of cause-and-effect. They can manifest themselves in symptoms that seem to have nothing to do with their causes, and they can appear or fail to appear in response to a whole web of circumstances, including the season, the weather, your diet, your state of mind, and the other allergy triggers in your environment. Under some circumstances, you might safely eat a food that, under other circumstances, will produce an adverse reaction. Or, there may be certain foods that, no matter what the circumstances, will inevitably set you coughing and choking.

## *Develop Your Awareness*

As a general principle, you should develop a sense of body awareness, a sensitivity to your own responses to food, weather, emotions, and your environment. Specifically, if you're concerned about allergies, keep an allergy journal. For two weeks keep a record of *everything* you eat and drink. At the end of each day, note how you felt during each between-meal period. Here's a sample page from Malcolm's food/allergy diary:

**Sample Food/Allergy Diary**

*Tuesday, July 14*

Woke up: 7 A.M.

| | |
|---|---|
| 7–9 A.M. | Felt generally good, a little foggy, a little tired |
| 9 A.M. | Coffee with cream and sugar, jelly donut (raspberry jelly) |
| 9 A.M.–1 P.M. | Pretty energetic until about 11 A.M., then felt a slight slump, nothing serious |
| 1 P.M. | Egg-salad sandwich on whole-wheat bread (mayonnaise, celery, egg, onion, salt, pepper, other?—ate in restaurant, not sure), french fries, coleslaw (with mayonnaise), chocolate cake with cream-cheese frosting, cola, coffee with cream and sugar |
| 1–3 P.M. | Felt bloated, gassy, tired, irritable |
| 3 P.M. | A few soda crackers, another cup of coffee, cream, sugar |
| 3–6:30 P.M. | More energetic, but still foggier than I was happy with, unsettled stomach |
| 6:30 P.M. | Chicken (no skin), baked potato, margarine, whole-wheat bread, cookies |
| 6:30–10:45 P.M. | Not so great, but better than this afternoon |
| 10:45 P.M. | Glass of skim milk, three store-bought chocolate-chip cookies |
| Bed: 11 P.M. | Slept reasonably well, but woke up twice during the night, once thought I was having another asthma attack, but I wasn't |

From the complete month-long diary the doctor might be able to suspect certain foods contributing to Malcolm's symptoms, whether allergic in etiology or not. For example, the chocolate cookies just before bed might have something to do with his sleep problems. (For more about diet, well-being, and asthma, see Chapter 8.)

## Elimination Diets

If you really want to find out whether food allergies are bringing down your overall level of vitality and effectiveness, you might try an elimination diet. Elimination diets are useful for two reasons: (1) Unlike allergy tests (which are discussed later in this chapter), elimination diets can help you discover very mild reactions to food. (2) Elimination diets are a dramatic way of discovering just how good you can feel when the allergy-causing foods are eliminated from your diet. However, if you are allergic to dust or other inhalants, you may not improve until those are also discovered and exposure is reduced.

The principle of an elimination diet is to eliminate all foods that you suspect are causing problems, to experience several trouble-free days, and then to gradually reintroduce "suspect" foods. If the newly introduced food produces symptoms with one challenge, it could be coincidence. However, if the symptom consistently follows the ingestion, that gives a strong suspicion of allergy.

*Caution*: Be sure to check with your doctor before starting an elimination diet, because if you eliminate a food and then reintroduce it, you might have a stronger reaction to it than you had when you were eating it continually. A doctor can help determine whether you have or are likely to have anaphylactic reactions to any food you are experimenting with. You should also religiously keep a food diary during any elimination diet, as both you and your doctor will be interested in your various reactions to this new way of eating.

The simplest elimination diet is to eliminate all junk foods for a week. If you feel a new burst of energy, if you're sleeping better, or if you notice fewer symptoms, you'll have found out something important about your diet!

If eliminating junk food doesn't make a dramatic difference, you might try eliminating the most common food allergens: cow's milk, wheat and wheat products, soy and soy products, and peanuts. If, after a week, you feel better, try reintroducing one food at a time, allowing yourself from two to seven days before reintroducing the next food. Try to reintroduce foods in their pure form: milk, rather than ice cream; cream of wheat, rather than bread; peanuts, rather than peanut butter. (For ideas on how to help children through an elimination diet, see Chapter 13.) Allergy testing can serve as a guide for an elimination trial diet. Allergy tests never "prove" the presence of clinical allergies, only that the IgE antibody is present.

If you'd like a more structured version of elimination diets, here are some suggestions:

## *Elimination Diet*

For one week, cut out all wheat, corn, yeast, eggs, dairy products, and soy products, such as soy sauce.

This is harder than it may sound, because

> Wheat is a filler in soups, cold cuts, lunch meats, and gravies.
> Yeast is used to make many vitamins, vinegars, pickles, malts, and alcoholic beverages, as well as in the mold used to age cheese (of course, you have already cut out dairy products!)
> Eggs are sometimes found in pasta.
> Milk is found in puddings, sauces, and some breads.

For this week, prepare and eat home-cooked foods as much as possible, concentrating on fresh fruits and vegetables, whole grains (rice, quinoa) and baked potatoes, fresh fish and chicken, and water and pure fruit juices.

Presumably, you or your family member will feel better after a week on this diet—if a bit bored by your food choices. Then you can reintroduce the eliminated foods one by one, giving each from two to three days. Most people start with the wheat since it is so difficult to avoid; then they add the milk, soy, or eggs. If your allergist/immunologist has tested you, the diet will be modified accordingly. The important thing is to remember not to stay on diets for prolonged periods unless there is good evidence of a reaction. Discuss this with your doctor.

## Food Families

If you have an adverse reaction to one particular food, it is possible that you may also react to others in the same "family"—a group of foods that share common genes. For example, if you are allergic to asparagus, which is in the lily family, you may also find that you are allergic to onions or another member of the lily family. This is known as cross-sensitivity. In most cases, you don't have to worry about related foods, but if you're noticing new adverse reactions, check the lists in Appendix B to find out if you've developed sensitivities to other foods in the family.

## Other Problem Foods

By now, you may have identified some foods that have been causing you problems. Or you may still be wondering how to identify your food allergies. Here are some more potential culprits. If any of these are your favorite foods, or foods that you eat often, consider eliminating them from your diet for a week or two and noting the results:

*Alcoholic Beverages* This category includes wine, beer, and hard liquor. Alcohol tends to cause blood to come rushing into the capillaries (a heavy drinker often has a red nose from the extra blood in those tiny blood vessels). You have a thick network of capillaries under the epithelium—the lining of the airways—and extra blood in the capillaries causes them to swell. Alcohol frequently accentuates absorption of foods. Beer and red wine also contain sulfites, additives that may provoke strong responses.

*Sulfites* These common preservatives are used in a wide variety of foods. They were once even used to preserve lettuce in salad bars, though that practice has stopped. Sulfite becomes sulfur dioxide gas, which, when inhaled, can irritate asthmatic lungs. Ironically, sulfur dioxide was once actually used in the nebulizers given to people with asthma and other lung diseases.

Sulfites may be found in processed potatoes, dried fruits and vegetables, chili mixes, prepared hashes and chowders, tomato sauce, syrups, prepared toppings and dips, potted cheese, processed cheeses, fruit juice, soft drinks, beer, wine, cider, vinegar, and pickles.

*Tartrazine* This yellow dye (FD&C yellow #5) may be found in a variety of processed foods that are yellow or orange, or even green or red. It may also be found in some medications that have been colored yellow or orange. People who are sensitive to aspirin occasionally have problems with tartrazine.

## Becoming a Food Detective

As Malcolm found out when he ordered the wild mushroom soup, it's not easy to avoid food allergens. Sometimes they are hidden and show up in foods we'd least suspect. Here's a list of foods to watch out for, in both home and restaurant cooking:

- *Tuna* sometimes contains "hydrolyzed plant protein," a flavor enhancer made from *soy*.
- *Turkey breast* includes filler that may have *wheat* (as well as fat).
- *Soy milk* may be sweetened with *barley malt*.
- *Cereal* may be sweetened with *barley malt* or with a *fermented sweetener*.
- *Crabmeat* is often imitation, made from *pollack (fish)* and enhanced with *artificial flavor and color*.
- *M&M's* are made with *peanuts*, even the plain ones!
- *Vitamins* are often made with *yeast*, *filler*, and *dyes*.

*Hidden Dangers* Many foods have hidden fats, sugars, and additives, which will not provoke an allergic reaction but which may not be healthful for you.

Restaurants can also pose pitfalls for allergic eaters. Many restaurant foods have "hidden ingredients" that even the servers may not be aware of. The waiter who failed to warn Malcolm about the canned chicken stock in the mushroom soup, for example, may not have known that the chef was taking such shortcuts.

*Creating a Healthy Diet* When you eat out, try to order foods that are prepared as simply as possible: baked or broiled fish, baked potato, salad with no dressing (lemon and olive oil on the side), fresh vegetables. Remember that mashed potatoes may have margarine or oil, soups may be made from prepared stock, and other foods may include one or more of the *2,000* commonly used additives in foods. Be especially wary of restaurant food if you are following an elimination diet.

## Triggers Not Found in Food

Not all triggers are found in food. Many are elsewhere in our home and work environments. (For a more complete discussion of environmental asthma triggers, see Chapters 6 and 7.) And some are medications. IgE antibodies may develop to medications, especially antibiotics, and cause mild or even severe allergic reactions. However, some medications can cause reactions by nonallergic (non-IgE) mechanisms. The following are such drugs.

### *Aspirin*

As many as one in every five people with asthma experience increased narrowing of the airways when they take aspirin or one of the so-called NSAIDs—nonsteroidal anti-inflammatory drugs. You are more likely to be sensitive to these medications if you have nasal polyps or chronic sinusitis in addition to your asthma. If you are being treated for headache, arthritis, or any type of chronic pain or inflammation, you may be taking one of the following medications:

    Aspirin and acetylsalicylic acid
    Diclofenac sodium (*Cataflam, Voltaren*)
    Etodolac (*Lodine*)
    Ibuprofen (*Advil, Motrin, Nuprin*)
    Ketoprofen (*Orudis$_{KT}$*)
    Indomethacin (*Indocin*)

Ketrolac (*Toradol*)
Meclofenamate (*Meclomen*)
Mefenamic acid (*Ponstel*)
Naproxen (*Naprosyn, Aleve, Anaprox*)
Nabumetone (*Relafen*)
Piroxicam (*Feldene*)
Sulindac (*Clinoril*)
Tolmetin (*Tolectin*)

Moreover, aspirin is an ingredient in many over-the-counter drugs—and new versions of NSAIDs are coming onto the market all the time. Discuss with your doctor your intake of aspirin or any medication—prescription or nonprescription—that you take for headache, arthritis, or inflammation. Even if you've been taking aspirin or a NSAID for years with no apparent ill effects, you should still talk it over with your physician. As mentioned earlier, allergic reactions can develop, apparently out of nowhere, after years of uneventful exposure.

### *Beta-Blockers*

This medication is given to people with high blood pressure, coronary heart disease, glaucoma, and headache. These drugs (whose full name is beta-adrenergic blocking agents) block impulses to the sympathetic nerves, which seems not to be a problem for people without asthma. However, the drugs do seem to make hyperresponsive airways more likely to close. Some people first discovered their asthmatic tendencies by having an adverse response to a beta-blocker; so again, if you are taking or considering taking one of the following medications, even in the form of eye drops, *talk it over with your doctor*:

Acebutolol (*Sectral*)
Atenolol (*Tenormin*)
Betaxolol (*Betopic*)
Betaxolol (*Kerlone*)

Bisoprolol (*Zebeta*)
Carteolol (*Cartol*)
Labetalol (*Normodyne*)
Labetalol (*Trandate*)
Metoprolol (*Lopressor*)
Metoprolol (*Toprol XL*)
Nadolol (*Corgard*)
Penbutolol (*Levatol*)
Pindolol (*Visken*)
Propranolol (*Inderal*)
Sotalol (*Betapace*)
Timolol (*Blocadren*)

***Angiotensin Converting Enzyme Inhibitors (Antihypertensive medication)***

Recent reports suggest that all the drugs in this class may potentiate an allergic reaction–they may allow a more severe reaction in insect sting patients. Cough is an occasional side effect, as is angioedema (swelling), especially of the tongue and upper airway. Examples of drugs in this group are Accupril, Lotensin, Monopril, Prinivil, Vasotec, Zestril, Altace, and Mavik. You should be sure your asthma physician is informed if you are on these medicines.

## Allergy Tests

If you and your doctor decide that allergies are a concern for you, your doctor may order one or more of a number of allergy tests. They may provide a guide for environmental changes, trial elimination diets, or immunotherapy in resistant cases.

*Skin Allergy Tests*   Here are the ones that doctors most commonly order:

- *Prick or puncture test*–The skin is pricked or punctured with an applicator on which a drop of allergen has been placed.

- *Intradermal test*—A small amount of allergen is injected under the skin. This method is used only *after* a prick test has been shown to be nonreactive.
- *Scratch test*—The skin is scratched with a "scarifier" and then a drop of allergen is placed on the skin. (Rarely used now.)

In any of these tests, if the skin develops a red wheal in fifteen to twenty minutes, that indicates IgE mediated sensitivity but does not by itself prove clinical allergy.

*Measuring Your IgE*  Your doctor may also try to determine how "allergic" you are overall by measuring your IgE levels. As explained earlier, IgE is the primary antibody that reacts to allergens, and it is highly provocative in promoting other inflammatory chemicals. People with asthma tend to have higher IgE levels than other people. Indeed, a 1992 study in the *New England Journal of Medicine* found that the higher your IgE levels, the more likely you are to have asthma, although some patients with normal levels of IgE in the bloodstream still test positive for allergies.

*RAST Tests*  Your doctor may order a RAST—radio absorbent test—to determine whether you have IgE antibodies to mold, dust, pollens, or certain foods. This method is used if you have extensive skin rash or are on a medication that blocks skin tests. Also, a few patients have severe reactions to skin testing; so if you have a history of anaphylaxis, your doctor may prefer to draw a blood sample and have it tested. This is somewhat less accurate than skin testing, but it is safer.

*Eosinophilia*  Eosinophils are cells that show up in your blood and tissues in the late stages of an inflammatory or allergic reaction. They help cause airways to narrow, and they seem to cause damage to the tissue that lines the lungs. A high concentration of eosinophils—which is what this test measures—indicates active asthma and probably damaged lung tissue. Your physician may examine your sputum or the secretions from your nose for presence of eosinophils.

## Becoming Aware

The importance of self-awareness in dealing with allergies cannot be stressed too often. First, however reliant you feel upon your doctor, in this area your doctor is highly reliant on *you*. Only you have—or can get—the detailed information about what you ate and inhaled, where you went and what you found there, how and when you reacted. All of this information can help your doctor discover what allergies you have and how severe they are.

Second, allergies are not always a simple cause-and-effect reaction. A substance that is harmful one day seems harmless the next, and vice versa. The degree of reaction may depend on the total allergic "load" in your body. For example, you may tolerate a certain level of exposure to dust mites until a pollen appears. Then you may react to both. Finally, your best guide is your own sense of what your body can handle, informed but not replaced by study and consultation with your doctor. So enjoy getting to know yourself and your body better! You may find that the process brings many benefits in addition to an easing of allergies and asthma.

*Ask Your Doctor ...*

- Should we be exploring an elimination diet?
- Should I be working with a nutritionist to explore diet, allergy, and asthma?
- Should I be working with an allergist, immunologist, or other specialist?
- What diet or lifestyle changes might help suppress or calm my allergies?
- What allergy tests do I need?
- What clues in my life lead you to suggest those tests?
- Do I show symptoms of food allergies?
- Do I need to be concerned about aspirin and other NSAIDs?
- Do I need to be concerned about taking beta-blockers?
- Do I need to be concerned about latex exposure?
- Would allergy shots help?

# 6

# Breathe Easier: Controlling Your Environment

Lydia's cough is getting worse and worse. She has stopped exercising, because she coughs and wheezes too much when she uses the treadmill. She used to enjoy a good game of tennis on the weekends, but now she has to stop and cough every time she exerts herself on the court. Lydia knows that the less she exercises, the less energy she has, but she doesn't know what to do. She is also feeling tired because the cough keeps waking her up at night, which interferes with her sleep.

When Lydia finally goes to see her doctor, he prescribes cough medicine for her, but that doesn't seem to do any good—and she starts to worry about taking too much cough medicine. Once again, she returns to her doctor.

Lydia's doctor performs some tests—and discovers that she does, in fact, have asthma. He begins to discuss with her the various types of asthma triggers, particularly those in her environment.

Now Lydia is more concerned than ever. Her doctor has told her that she may become ever more sensitive to all sorts of factors in her environment, at home, in other indoor environments, and outdoors. After talking with her doctor, Lydia worries that she may develop hay fever, allergic reactions to pollen, sensitivity to wood smoke, intolerance of mold, or reactions to household chemicals.

Lydia can't imagine how she can possibly avoid all of these potential triggers. She wants to lead a normal life—

but she certainly doesn't want to get any sicker. What should she do?

## You Are What You Breathe

Lydia has just found out the truth of this slogan in a particularly personal way: suddenly, the very air she breathes seems to be affecting every aspect of her life! Yet understanding the role of environment in her asthma will help Lydia manage her symptoms and create a workable approach to her health.

Recall that the purpose of breathing is to take air from your environment and put it into your body. True, your body is only interested in extracting oxygen from the air, but you can't get the oxygen without taking in all the rest of your immediate atmosphere as well. Your lungs and nose purify the air a little bit, as the cilia in nasal passages and airways attempt to catch many of the particles or foreign matter that you might breathe in. Still, there is much in the air that is far too small to be stopped by your cilia, such as pollen fragments, mold spores, dust mites, chemical fumes, and smoke.

An adult breathes in fifteen times a minute; a child, even more often. For adults, that's 600 breaths an hour, or over 12,000 breaths a day. Or think of it this way: we inhale a pint of air fifteen times a minute. That's 22,000 pints of air a day. Think of all the pollen, mold spores, dust, chemical fumes, and other foreign matter that we are taking into our bodies with each breath—and multiply that by 12,000 breaths or 22,000 pints!

People who don't have asthma generally don't even notice all the particles they breathe in—but people who do have asthma notice far more than they would like. Their inflamed, hyperresponsive airways react in two ways: with allergic reactions, which, as explained in Chapter 4, set off an inflammatory cascade of chemicals; and with irritation, which can cause the overly sensitive bronchial lining to react and provoke a bronchospasm.

This chapter looks at the kinds of environmental factors—material that is breathed in—that can cause problems for people with asthma: outdoor allergens and household allergens and irritants. Each section discusses both the dangers and some ways to minimize, avoid, or eliminate them. (For more information on workplace hazards and air pollution, see Chapter 7.)

## The Great Outdoors

The primary outdoor allergens are plant pollens and mold spores. Let's look at each in turn.

### *Plant Pollens*

In the past, it was relatively simple to identify different types of pollen with different parts of the United States. This regional specificity made it easier for people with asthma to identify their particular "hot spots" and, perhaps, to avoid them.

Now, however, pollens have migrated across the country, so that it is far harder for people with asthma to identify "safe" areas. Moreover, pollen counts have risen in many, if not all, parts of the United States. This is a human-made phenomenon: suburban development brings with it lawns, shade trees, and golf courses, all of which produce pollen. In Fresno, California, for example, one doctor estimated that pollen counts were rising by 15 percent a year, as housing with Bermuda grass lawns and mulberry trees has proliferated in local housing tracts. The city of Tucson, Arizona, has banned mulberry trees and instituted fines against homeowners who let Bermuda grass grow too high.

How can you tell whether you have pollen allergies? Here's some information that may help you decide:

- Pollen counts are usually highest in the mornings.
- Clear and windy days tend to make pollen allergies worse (because the wind blows around more pollen).
- After the first frost, pollen allergies tend to clear up.
- During rain, pollen allergies tend to clear up or at least to temporarily subside a bit.
- Air conditioning helps mitigate allergies to pollen.

If you do suffer from pollen allergies, you need to know which trees, grasses, and weeds are in bloom when. The following lists are arranged by season and by region, but keep in mind that pollen migrates.

**Tree Pollen Seasons**

*Desert Southwest, Including Texas*

*Oak*–March–June
*Mesquite*–March–June
*Cottonwood*–February–April

*Intermountain Region*

*Oak*–May–June
*Birch*–April–June
*Cottonwood/Poplar*–
  March–May
*Maple/Box Elder*–
  April–May

*Northeast/Central United States*

*Oak*–April–June
*Birch*–April–June
*Cottonwood/Poplar*–
  March–May
*Maple/Box Elder*–
  February–May

*Pacific Northwest*

*Oak*–April–June
*Black Walnut*–April–May
*Chinese Elm*–
  February–April
*Alder*–February–March

**Grass Pollen Seasons**

*Desert Southwest, Including Texas*

*Bermuda*–April–November
*Brome*–May–July
*June (Kentucky Blue)*–April–July
*Sudan Grass*–May–October

*Intermountain Region*

*Timothy*–May–August
*Orchard*–May–July
*June (Kentucky Blue)*–
  May–July
*Brome*–May–September

*Northeast/Central United States*

*Timothy*–May–August
*Orchard*–May–July
*June (Kentucky Blue)*–
  May–July
*Red Top*–May–July

*Pacific Northwest*

*Timothy*–April–August
*Orchard*–April–July
*Italian Rye*–April–August
*June (Kentucky Blue)*–
  April–September
*Brome*–April–September

| Southeast and South Central United States | Southeast and South Central United States |
|---|---|
| *Cedar/Elm*–February–March | *Bermuda*–February–December |
| *Oak*–April–May | *Johnson*–May–October |
| *Birch*–April–May | *June (Kentucky Blue)*– May–June |
| *Pecan*–April–May | |
| *Maple/Box Elder*– February–May | *Timothy*–May–July |
| | *Orchard*–May–June |

There's not much you can do directly about pollen allergies except to stay indoors, preferably in an air-conditioned environment, during the times that your particular pollen allergen is at its highest count. You can also begin preventive medication before the pollen appears. However, with attention to other environmental factors as well as to the types of overall health improvement discussed in Chapters 8 and 9, you may be able to calm your system down to the point where you become far less responsive to pollen allergens. Allergen immunotherapy (allergy shots) are very effective in reducing sensitivity to pollen.

## *Molds*

In the autumn, when damp leaves pile up on lawns or in gutters, mold spores float through the air to plague the lungs of people with asthma. So people who have both asthma and mold allergies have good reason to see fall as their most difficult season. However, molds can proliferate at any time of year, even in winter.

How can you tell if you are allergic to mold? If you answer yes to one or more of the following questions, you may have a mold allergy that you should discuss further with your doctor:

- Are your allergies less bothersome when temperatures are below freezing?
- Are you more comfortable at the ocean's edge or in the desert, where molds are less likely to grow? Correspondingly, are you less comfortable in the country, the suburbs, and small towns?
- Do you have asthma symptoms after raking leaves?

- Do you feel worse outdoors at night? (Molds flourish in the evening, whereas the hot, bright sun tends to discourage their growth.)
- Do you feel worse on rainy, humid days? (Molds thrive in damp conditions.)
- Do you have asthma symptoms in the autumn, after ragweed and other pollen seasons have ended? (In the South, ragweed lasts until November's frost–do your symptoms persist past that time?)
- Do your symptoms flare in musty places like basements and closets?

*What Can You Do about Outdoor Allergens?*

- Stay indoors when allergens are highest in the air; check with the weather service for information.
- Avoid long walks outside in the morning if you have pollen allergies, or in the evening if you have mold allergies.
- During your "problem seasons," keep your windows shut and rely on a good air conditioner with high-quality filters.
- Discuss with your doctor whether allergy shots are indicated.
- See Chapters 8 and 9 for suggestions on calming and restoring your immune system and Chapter 12 for information on preventive medications.

## Indoor Hazards

The major indoor asthma allergens are animal dander, dust mites, cockroaches, and indoor molds. Some of these are easier to eliminate from your home than others, but virtually every U.S. home is subject to at least one of these asthma triggers, and many homes are subject to all of them.

Consider, for example, that ideally, air would circulate throughout your home at the rate of 2.5 times an hour–every hour, you would have two and a half complete changes of air–as opposed to most homes' actual figure of only a 10 percent change in the home's air every hour. Recall that many homes today are carpeted—and then consider that cat dander can linger in a carpet for up to twenty-four weeks after the cat has gone. It is suggested that modern insulated homes, wall-to-wall carpeting, and increased numbers of indoor pets have all contributed to the rise in asthma.

## *Identifying Home-Based Allergens*

How can you tell if you or your family members have home-based allergies? These questions may help you decide:

- Are your allergies worse when you first wake up? Do you sleep on a feather pillow or use a feather comforter?
- Are your allergies worse during certain months? (This might indicate that you are reacting more to outdoor allergens, such as pollens and outdoor mold spores, although your timing might also correspond to periods when dust mites and indoor molds are at their height.)
- Do your allergies seem worse when you let the pets come indoors?
- Do you get allergic reactions or asthma symptoms after handling a pet?
- Does vacuuming give you asthma symptoms?
- Does making a bed give you asthma symptoms? Are there feather pillows in your home?
- Does being in the basement give you asthma symptoms? (This suggests that you might be reacting to mold.)
- Is there any particular activity that seems to give you asthma symptoms?
- Do you generally feel better at work or at home?
- When did you move into your home? What relationship does that have with the progression of your asthma symptoms?
- Do you feel better or worse when doors and windows are open? Closed?
- Do you have symptoms that disappear when you leave home?

Consider your answers to these questions, then take a look at the following information about common household allergens/asthma triggers. If you think you are allergic to any of these triggers, take some of the actions described below—and discuss the matter with your doctor.

*Animal Dander* Some 43 percent of all U.S. residents own dogs; 28 percent have cats; and 2 percent have rodents as pets. *All* domesticated mammals produce allergens—as do birds and other warm-blooded creatures. Cat allergen remains airborne for hours after a cat has been removed. It has even been detected in schools where cats have never been—but where the allergen has been brought in on children's clothing.

*Dust Mites* As their name suggests, these microscopic creatures live in dust. They eat animal dander, feathers, the flakes of skin shed by warm-blooded mammals—including humans, by the way. The particles may be dissolved and absorbed, causing asthma or allergic reactions.

The mites leave their waste products all over a house: in mattresses, pillows, bedcovers, furniture, carpeting, clothing, and soft toys. (The technical names for dust mites in North America are *Dermatophagoides farinae* and *D. pteronyssinus*, by the way.)

The fecal pellets are so small that you can fit 250,000 of them into a gram of household dust. They may trigger symptoms by settling in the nose or even penetrating into the lower airways at times.

Dust mites can live all year round in all homes, not just centrally heated ones, though they tend to peak in July and August, with lowest levels in April and May. Yet many dust mite–allergic people have symptoms worsened in the fall when the heat is first turned on. Some particles fly around as the air is dried by the heat. They can't live in altitudes above 5,000 feet, so you won't find them in Denver, Santa Fe, or other mountain regions. They're fairly common just about everywhere else, though.

*Cockroaches* Roach parts themselves are allergenic. Frequently, they mix with animal hair and mite pellets to make an allergenic triple threat. (Animal hair itself isn't allergenic, but it carries animal saliva and dander, which does provoke allergies.)

Because asthma rates are rising so dramatically among poor people, some scientists wonder about the relationship of poor living conditions–roach-infested houses and apartments–to the rise in asthma.

*Indoor Molds* Molds flourish in dark, humid, and poorly ventilated areas of a home: in the basement, kitchen, and bathroom, and in foam pillows. Mold also lives in air conditioners that can circulate spores throughout a home unless they are equipped with the proper filters. Humidifiers and dehumidifiers may contain reservoirs that promote mold growth.

## *What Can You Do about Home-based Asthma Triggers?*

### *Animals*

- Find another home for your pet. This is a hard decision, but remember, there's no such thing as a "nonallergenic" furry animal. Short hair doesn't solve the problem, because it's the animal's saliva and dander that carries the allergen, and saliva can mix with hair of any length or with dander (flakes of dead skin) to penetrate into your environment.
- If you do find another home for your pet, you still have to deal with the leftover allergen in your own home. A commercially available 3 percent tannic acid solution might help neutralize the remaining allergens.
- If you must keep the family pet, you might try keeping it out of the allergic person's bedroom.
- Seal up your home's air ducts, if you have forced-air heating, and use portable room heaters instead. That way, the animal allergen won't be passed from room to room by the heating system.
- Wash your pet once a week.

### *Dust Mites*

- Encase your mattress and pillow in an airtight cover. Many varieties now available do not sound noisy or promote sweating. The extra cost may be worthwhile because they last for several years.

- Wash your bedding weekly, in temperatures of at least 130°F. Because setting water heaters that high might be dangerous for children, some experts recommend keeping the bedding in the dryer for a longer time after washing instead.
- Don't sleep on upholstered furniture, even for short naps—or cover the furniture with a sheet or throw cover.
- Get rid of the bedroom carpet (because carpets are more hospitable to dust mites than bare floors are). If you can't remove the carpet, at least avoid sitting or lying on it without first putting a sheet or quilt on the floor.
- Reduce indoor humidity to below 50 percent, using a dehumidifier or air conditioner if necessary (but make sure your air conditioner is equipped with a special high-efficiency particulate air [HEPA] filter—and make sure you keep your filters clean!).
- Use appropriate chemicals to kill mites (talk to your doctor about this, as you don't want to use any chemical to which you may also be sensitive).
- When you travel, check the pillows and ask for non-feather ones.

*Cockroaches*

- Use an exterminator.
- Don't leave food out in the kitchen or anywhere else. Seal it in roach-proof containers.
- Explore various nontoxic antiroach devices, such as baking soda.
- Seal up areas around pipes under the sink where roaches might enter.

*Indoor Molds*

- Discover and eliminate any places that water is leaking or seeping into your home.
- Scrape, plaster, and repaint any mildewed or moldy places in your home.

- Use a dehumidifier, if necessary, to keep home humidity below 50 percent. Fans in the windows in laundry rooms, kitchens, and bathrooms can help ventilation. Be sure that the clothes dryer is vented properly to the outside.
- Make sure that all dehumidifiers, air conditioners, furnaces, freezers, and refrigerators are kept clean, particularly their evaporation trays and drains. Make sure that refrigerator seals are firm and work properly. Keep drip pans clean as well.
- Clean and disinfect shower tiles and kitchen counters at least once a week.

*General Tips*

- Consider getting a home air filter. These have some effectiveness against cigarette smoke (which shouldn't be in your house anyway; see the following section), mold spores, animal dander, and household dust. You might get a mechanical cleaner that uses a HEPA filter, or one that uses an electrostatic precipitator, which uses a static charge on metal plates to attract dust. You can buy free-standing room-sized units or ones that you can install in central heating or air-conditioning systems. *However, air filters don't substitute for other forms of allergen control.*
- If possible, people with asthma should avoid vacuuming (it stirs up too much dust), or at least, they should wear a face mask while doing this chore.
- Equip your vacuum cleaner with a HEPA filter or double bags to reduce dust emission.
- Avoid using a humidifier, which is a favorite home for molds and mites; or, if you must use one, make sure that you keep it clean.
- Using an air conditioner allows you to keep the windows closed, which shuts out outdoor pollens and lowers the humidity in your home, making it less hospitable to molds and mites.

## *Irritants*

What's the difference between an irritant and an allergen? An allergen triggers an adverse reaction only in someone who has a particular allergy. An irritant, on the other hand, bothers everybody—but only people who have asthma respond with asthma symptoms.

How can you tell if your asthma is responding to household irritants? Consider these questions:

- Have you recently purchased a new gas appliance, furnace, or stove? A new carpet? Drapes? Furniture?
- Have you recently dry-cleaned your drapes or clothes?
- Have you recently had your carpet or furniture cleaned?
- Have you recently used cleaning solvents, varnish, wood strippers, paints, glues, stains, or similar products?
- Have you recently done any remodeling or repairs, or had that work done for you?

If you have asthma and are bothered by any of the irritants discussed in this section, take heart. The irritants referred to here are the toxic substances that cause health problems, subtle or overt, for every human being who has heavy exposure to them.

*Cigarette Smoke* Tobacco smoke is one of the most common air pollutants—and one of the most deadly to *anyone.* But if you or a member of your family has asthma, your first step in avoiding attacks is quite simple: Keep tobacco smoke in all its forms entirely out of your home.

For at least half a century, people with asthma and their physicians have been aware of the negative effects of tobacco smoke, which has been linked to lung and heart disease, cancer, and general ill-health as well as to asthma. The specific toxic effects of tobacco smoke on people with asthma, however, make smoking a particularly deadly habit—dangerous to indulge in oneself or to be in the vicinity of someone who is smoking.

Tobacco smoke actually paralyzes the ciliated cells with hair-like projections that line the airways. For the body to stay healthy, the airways must clean themselves out, expelling the mucus and debris that our lungs accumulate every day. If the airway cilia are paralyzed, however, they can't perform this cleansing function. Not only does mucus build up in the lungs, it may also contribute to secondary infections.

Moreover, the poisonous carbon monoxide to be found in tobacco smoke irritates the lungs further, sometimes even to the point of collapse. The air sacs (alveoli) of a person with asthma are already in a fragile condition; contact with irritating smoke can weaken them even more. Besides the carbon monoxide, cigarettes contain more than two hundred known poisons, including benzene and formaldehyde.

In recent years, a great deal of attention has been focused on the role of secondhand smoke in causing lung disease. While this is still a controversial topic with regard to many ailments, the dangers of secondhand smoke to people with asthma are unmistakable. Children who live in homes where parents smoke, for example, are hospitalized for asthma more frequently and have longer hospital stays than do children who live in homes where no one smokes.

*Formaldehyde* Used chiefly as a preservative and a disinfectant and as an aid in the combining of chemicals, formaldehyde is an invisible but pungent irritating gas–and sometimes an asthma trigger.

Some 6 billion pounds of formaldehyde are manufactured in the United States each year, to be used in oil-based paints, soft plastics (such as shower curtains), fabrics, paper towels, grocery bags, detergents, toiletries, cosmetics, and many other products. Formaldehyde and furniture are related: Consider that particleboard, a popular building material, is made of wood chips held together by glues and resins that can emit formaldehyde gas. After carpet or particleboard is aired for a couple of hours, the emitting of formaldehyde usually drops to levels that are not bothersome.

*Nitrogen Dioxide and Carbon Dioxide* When fuel is burned in gas stoves, furnaces, boilers, and kerosene heaters, nitrogen dioxide is released. This gas can irritate the eyes, nose, and throat, can interfere with the lungs' ability to function, and can trigger respiratory infections. Nitrogen dioxide at high levels can cause a person with asthma to suffer from shortness of breath, coughing, headaches, and increased mucus production.

Excessive amounts of carbon dioxide is found in homes (and offices) that are not properly ventilated, when the air that humans exhale builds up in the enclosed atmosphere. Headaches, dizziness, increased heart rate, and high blood pressure are only some of the symptoms that can result from living or working in poorly ventilated air.

*Pesticides*  Did you know that the first modern pesticide had its origin in the 1940s, as a nerve gas developed by Germany for use in World War II? No wonder the fumes from these now-common chemicals can irritate the eyes, nose, throat, and lungs. If you use pesticides in your garden, handle them with care, making sure to wear appropriate clothing and a mask.

*Volatile Chemicals*  Chemicals of this type are found in many common household products, such as ammonia, acetic acid, benzene, acetone, ethanol, methanol, and the like. Cleaners, shampoos, disinfectants, solvents, sealants, aerosol sprays, air fresheners, paint thinners, paint removers, and similar products frequently contain volatile chemicals–whose irritating fumes can endanger people both with and without asthma. Long-term heavy exposure to such chemical fumes can sensitize the lungs to other toxins. Even short-term exposure can irritate the throat and lungs, while making the eyes and nose burn. In some cases, people feel nauseous or dizzy, or develop headache or chest pain.

Paint is a major source of chemical fumes. That's why people with asthma often suffer reactions to newly painted homes or workplaces. Oil-based paints contain some thirty to forty volatile chemicals, whereas water-based paints contain twelve to fifteen, plus biocides. Although biocides do prevent mold from growing, they can also trigger asthma in some people.

*Wood Smoke*  What could be more romantic than a wood fire, more comforting than the smell of a wood-burning stove? Unfortunately, some people with asthma may have strong reactions to wood smoke. The smoke may trigger an asthmatic reaction, particularly when wood is burned in a poorly ventilated area, such as an insulated home during winter.

*Perfumes and Other Strong Scents* Perfume, cosmetics, room deodorants, insect repellents, and other strongly scented items may provoke an asthmatic reaction. It's possible that the reaction is caused by the chemicals used to create the scent, or it may be a by-product of the body's attempt to avoid the smell.

## What Can You Do to Avoid Irritants?

### Smoke

- Quit smoking, and get everyone who lives in your home to do the same.
- Refuse to allow any visitor, whether social guests or repair and delivery people, to smoke in your home.
- Don't ride in a car in which anyone is smoking, even if all the windows are open.
- Commit to finding smoke-free public places. If a restaurant or other establishment has only a tiny, overcrowded no-smoking section, or a no-smoking area that is overwhelmed by smoke from the neighboring smoking section, avoid that place or explain to the manager the health problems that such an arrangement poses for you (or your child).
- Don't allow your child to be cared for in an area where smoking is allowed.

### Formaldehyde

- Remove synthetic carpets and replace them with either hardwood floors or washable, removable rugs if possible.
- Avoid particleboard and fiberboard when you build or buy products, or try to air out areas where they are used for several days. Note that medium-density fiberboard (MDF) emits almost three times as much formaldehyde as particleboard.

### Nitrogen Dioxide and Carbon Dioxide

- Monitor your fuel-burning appliances to see if they release these gases. (You can buy simple devices to do this.)

- Do everything you can to ventilate the rooms in which you live and work. Make sure that all fuel-burning appliances are in properly ventilated areas.

*Pesticides*

- If possible, avoid chemical pesticides; use natural ones instead.
- If you must use pesticides, wash thoroughly after working with them; if possible, wear protective gloves, glasses, and breathing masks.

*Volatile Chemicals*

- Make sure that any room in which painting takes place is well ventilated.
- Use care when opening a dishwasher when it is running, because the hot steam will contain detergent.
- Don't use scented candles, sprays, or potpourri.

## Coping with Environmental Changes

At first glance, the information in this chapter may seem well-nigh overwhelming. You may be wondering if there is *any* aspect of your environment that you don't have to worry about.

In any case, start by looking at *every* aspect of your environment, if only to discover both potential and actual triggers for your asthma attacks. Many environmental changes are relatively easy to make—and making these changes may so reduce the number of stresses on your system that you won't be faced with making the more difficult alterations.

Even if you do have to take some radical steps—removing the wall-to-wall carpeting, giving away the family pet—take heart. Consult with your doctor or allergist to develop a workable plan for making changes. Continue to address the issues of diet, exercise, and breathing exercises, as described in the other chapters of this book. Change is a long, slow process—but as your asthma symptoms decrease and your health improves, you may find that it is a rewarding process as well.

## Ask Your Doctor...

- What outdoor allergens am I reacting to?
- Are there particular times of day that I should try to stay indoors?
- What problems am I encountering in my home environment?
- How can I find out more about what health hazards might be in my home?
- What steps can I take to make my home a safer place for me?
- What priorities should I set about making changes at home? What elements seem to be causing the worst or the most immediate problems?
- Is it worth it for me to invest in an air filter?
- Do we have to give away the family pet? Is there another alternative?
- Do I have to get rid of the wall-to-wall carpeting? Is there another alternative?
- What sources of formaldehyde in my home may be causing me trouble?
- Although everyone in my household has stopped smoking, our relatives still smoke, and I hate to tell them they can't. I'm willing to ask them not to smoke in our home, but what should I do about visits to theirs?
- Would allergy shots help to decrease my level of sensitivity?

# 7

# Occupational Hazards and Air Pollution

Lydia is still puzzled about how she developed asthma and why it seemed to come on so suddenly. Then someone at work says that she's heard of bakery workers contracting asthma from breathing in all the flour dust. Lydia does some research about workplace-related health hazards–and discovers a disease that she'd never heard of before: occupational asthma, which you get in response to conditions at work. Her doctor confirms that indeed, occupational asthma is what she has.

This information makes Lydia both frustrated and angry. She's angry because she hates the idea that the very work she does to earn a living is so dangerous to her health. She's frustrated, because she seems to have two equally upsetting choices–to quit her job or to continue getting sicker.

As Lydia learns more, she develops some new concerns. Now she worries that her newly sensitive lungs may react with asthma symptoms whenever air pollution in her city is particularly heavy. How can she cope with this new health hazard?

## Workplace Hazards

How common is Lydia's problem–and what can she do about it?

Some 2 percent of all the people in the United States–that's one person in every fifty–suffer from workplace exposure to irritants and allergens. Occupational asthma affects up to 10 percent of those who work with lab animals, and, according to the National Bureau of Health Statistics, up to 40 percent of those who work in small bakeries, like Lydia. As in Lydia's case, occupational asthma can be a slow-acting disease that appears only after weeks or even years of exposure.

### *Identifying the Problem*

Are you suffering from occupational asthma? Consider these questions:

- Are your symptoms worse at work or just after you come home?
- Do your symptoms tend to clear up on weekends and vacations?
- Even if your symptoms now seem constant, did they once follow this pattern?

A wide variety of occupations seems to threaten people with occupational asthma. We provide a brief list here, but if your occupation isn't on the list, don't assume that you are exempt. Work with your doctor to determine whether your symptoms are stemming from work.

**Occupational Asthma Triggers**

| Occupation | Agent |
|---|---|
| *Animal Sources* | |
| Veterinarians, lab animal workers | Animal dander, urine |
| Food processors/ pharmaceutical workers | Shellfish, egg proteins, pancreatic enzymes, amylase |
| Dairy farmers | Storage mites |
| Poultry farmers | Poultry mites, droppings, feathers |
| Granary workers | Storage mites, aspergillus, indoor ragweed, grass pollen |

| | |
|---|---|
| Detergent manufacturing | *Bacillus subtilis* enzymes |
| Silk workers | Silkworm moths and larvae |

*Plant Sources*

| | |
|---|---|
| Bakers | Flour |
| Food processors | Coffee bean dust, meat tenderizer (papain), tea |
| Farmers | Soybean dust |
| Shipping workers | Grain dust (molds, insects, grains) |
| Sawmill workers, carpenters, pulp workers, bark strippers, cork workers | Wood dust—western red cedar, oak, mahogany, zebrawood, redwood, cedar, African maple, eastern white cedar |
| Electric soldering | Colophony (pine resin) |
| Cotton textile workers | Cotton dust (which produces so-called mill fever) |
| Nurses | Psyllium, latex |

*Inorganic Chemical Sources*

| | |
|---|---|
| Refining | Platinum salts |
| Plating | Nickel salts |
| Diamond polishing | Cobalt salts |
| Stainless steel welding | Chromium salts |
| Manufacturing | Aluminum fluoride |
| Hair styling | Persulfate |
| Refinery workers | Vanadium |
| Welding | Stainless steel fumes |

*Organic Chemical Sources*

| | |
|---|---|
| Manufacturing | Antibiotics, piperzaine, methyl-dopa, salbutanol, cimetidine |
| Hospital workers | Disinfectants (sulfathiazole, chloramine, formaldehyde, glutaraldehyde) |
| Anesthesiology | Enflurane |
| Fur dyeing | Paraphenylene diamine |

| | |
|---|---|
| Rubber processing | Formaldehyde, ethylene diamine, phthalic anhydride |
| Plastics manufacturing | Toluene diisocyanate, hexamethyl diisocyanate, diphenylmethyl diisocyanate, phthalic anhydride, triethylene tetramines, trimellitic anhydride, hexamethyl tetramine |
| Automobile painting | Dimethyl ethanolamine, toluene diisocyanate |
| Foundry workers | Furfuryl alcohol resin |

## *Who Is at Risk?*

In general, anyone who works with latex, resins, metals, dyes, drugs, animals, or insects is at risk for occupational asthma. Here are some additional categories of workers who may be affected by workplace hazards:

- Aeronautical engineers, who work with thinners, solvents, anticorrosives, latex, formaldehyde, acrylic glues
- Artists, designers, decorators, painters, and refinishers, who work with acrylics, resins, pigments, thinners, solvents, polishes
- Auto mechanics, who work with brake fluid, gasoline, cleansers, chromium, anticorrosive paints, nickel
- Pharmacists and physicians, who work with antibiotics and latex gloves

## *Building-Related Illnesses*

What about people who work primarily with paper, telephones, and computers–that is, people who work in offices? Are they also at risk from occupational asthma?

The answer is yes. First of all, offices are built and renovated with the same materials as homes are. They, too, are carpeted with products that emit formaldehyde, and they may be painted with oil-based paint. (Remember how Malcolm's symptoms got worse after he moved into his new office?) Likewise, offices may be cleaned with industrial cleaners that release fumes, and some are heated and cooled by central systems that fail to provide the desired 2.5 air changes per hour. Poorly ventilated offices are high in levels of carbon monoxide. Photocopiers give off ozone, a toxin and an irritant; other office equipment may also do so. Even the innocuous bottle of white-out may release fumes that trigger an asthmatic attack.

The term "building-related illness" has recently come into use. This term is used when buildings in which some 20 percent of the occupants have adverse reactions because of environmental problems within the building.

### *Canary in the Coal Mine*

Once again, the image of the canary in the coal mine comes to mind. Miners concerned about loss of oxygen or dangerous fumes in the mine shaft would bring a caged canary into the mine shaft with them. If the bird died, they knew they were in danger.

Likewise, people with asthma seem to react first and most intensely to the conditions that are causing problems for everyone else around them. This sensitivity is a double-edged sword; on the one hand, the ever-present threat of illness can be discouraging to people with asthma. On the other, that very threat means that they may be taking better care of their health than people without asthma, who are also being subjected to toxins, irritants, and insults to the lungs on a daily basis.

## Protecting Your Work Environment

How can you make sure that you are working in a safe and healthy environment? Although workplaces are supposed to be inspected regularly by the Occupational Health and Safety Administration (OSHA), the average workplace is now inspected only once every eighty-four years. That puts the responsibility for monitoring their workplaces on employees themselves. It's now up to you and your co-workers to ensure your own safety, working with your employer and your physician to eliminate workplace health hazards.

### *What Can You Do to Avoid Workplace Health Hazards?*

- Educate yourself. Work with your building superintendent, with your employee health physician, with other workplace health-and-safety organizations, and with your co-workers to find out what kinds of health hazards you might be encountering at work.
- Wear whatever protective clothing, masks, and other safety devices are provided. If the proper protective devices aren't available, work to have them provided for you and your co-workers.
- Poorly ventilated offices and businesses can often be helped by bringing in plants, which release oxygen.
- It may be possible to make other arrangements for your office if you are having trouble with the central air-conditioning or heating systems. For example, you may be able to use a room-size HEPA filter. Explore these possibilities with building management.
- It may be possible to transfer to another type of job at your workplace, one that doesn't involve exposure to allergens or irritants. Find out what your company's rules are, and work with the company doctor as well as with your personal physician.

## **Air Pollution and Industrial Development**

As shown in this and earlier chapters, the main asthma triggers seem to be found in indoor air, in homes and offices. Certainly the industrial development that has flooded our lives with chemicals may be related to the rise of asthma and asthma-related deaths in the last two decades. But air pollution of various types triggers asthmatic reactions, even if it is not directly responsible for the rise in new cases of asthma. Moreover, in some locations—particularly in poor neighborhoods around wood- and coal-burning factories, and in poor neighborhoods in Los Angeles—air pollution may be more of a culprit than elsewhere. Yet, as auto exhaust pollution has been reduced, the severity of asthma has increased.

*Acid Rain* Sulfur and nitrogen dioxide are produced by burning wood and coal. These gases combine with water droplets to form sulfuric and nitric acids, popularly known as acid rain. Possibly these gases behave the same way within our airways, combining with mucus to form a kind of corrosive acidic mucus. At the very least, this would irritate the lungs of people with asthma. At most, it might make the difference between developing and not developing asthma.

*Long-Term Damage* Part of the problem with trying to evaluate the role of air pollution in asthma (and allergy) is that no one knows what the long-term effects on our airways might be. The effects of pollution may be gradual, subtle, and not immediately apparent—until they later show up as vulnerability to asthma and allergy.

For example, one study of an integrated steel mill in the Utah Valley found that hospital admissions for asthma for preschoolers was two times greater than that of a neighboring valley, which had only half the particulate pollution. This was true even though the less polluted, less asthmatic valley had higher rates of smoking and lower temperatures (cold air can trigger asthma). Moreover, twice the number of children were hospitalized for asthma when the steel mill was operating than when it was not.

*Social Conditions* In the United States, class and race are closely bound up with where people live—and how healthy they are. In March 1990, Dr. Russell Sherwin, a University of Southern California pathologist, performed autopsies on a hundred youths who had died either in accidents or in homicides. Most of the young people he autopsied were African American and Latino youth of South Central Los Angeles, an impoverished neighborhood. Dr. Sherwin found that some 27 percent had "severe lesions" on their lungs, and 80 percent had "notable lung abnormalities ... above and beyond what we've seen with smoking or even respiratory viruses ..." He believed that if these young people had lived, they would have had clinical lung disease by age forty.

*Synergy* As with other asthma triggers, synergy can make hyperresponsive lungs ever more sensitive. One irritant or allergen can start the lungs off on a cycle that produces ever more inflammation and sensitivity, so that progressively more factors—both irritants such as paint fumes and harmless substances such as cat dander—trigger an asthmatic response. Certainly, air pollution may be lowering the threshold of sensitivity, so to speak, particularly in the poor neighborhoods where industrial waste and factory emissions are at their highest.

### *Short- and Long-Term Approaches*

What does this mean for someone trying to deal with the day-to-day realities of asthma? It means that there may be two tracks on which to address the problem: the immediate effort to clean up your own environment at home and at work, and the long-term attempt to clean up the environment in which we all live. There is definitely a great deal you can do to control the spaces in which you personally spend the most time. There is also much you can do to address the problems of the larger environment. When thinking about how to cope with your asthma, keep both arenas in mind!

### *Ask Your Doctor ...*

- Are my asthma symptoms work-related?
- How can I find out more about which symptoms are work-related?
- What steps should I be taking to make work a safer place for me?
- At what level of smog alert should I begin to be concerned?
- Is there somewhere in the city where I can get a more specific and frequent reading of local smog levels?

# 8

# Nourishing Your Mind, Body, and Spirit: A Holistic Approach

Malcolm is so concerned about the number of food allergies he seems to have developed that he begins working with a nutritionist. The nutritionist looks at Malcolm's food diary and shakes her head. "Even if you didn't have asthma," she says, "this diet would make you feel tired and groggy." She asks Malcolm if he's willing to experiment with other ways of eating, just for two weeks or a month. At that point, she says, if he feels better, he can decide for himself if he wants to go back to his old way of eating. Malcolm agrees to take her suggestions.

The nutritionist puts Malcolm on a low-fat diet with lots of whole grains and fresh vegetables. Malcolm tells her that he loves coffee and desserts, so they work out some limits: one cup of coffee in the morning and one after lunch, but with two-percent milk instead of cream; "real" desserts three times a week, with fresh fruit the rest of the time. The nutritionist also asks Malcolm to avoid any kinds of additives or preservatives, and because he seems to have a mild allergy to them, to avoid eggs as well.

Sure enough, within two weeks, Malcolm is sleeping better and feeling more rested. And within a month, Malcolm not only has more energy, but he also seems to be far less sensitive to allergens. Malcolm has mixed feelings: he misses his old way of eating and finds the new way a lot more trouble (fewer restaurants, fewer treats)—but he does love his new sense of health and well-being.

Angela believes that the mind and the body are connected, so she starts to think about her emotional state and how it might relate to her asthma. She begins to keep a book that she calls her "Asthma Journal," in which she writes three pages each day. When she first started keeping the journal, Angela just wrote about asthma—what she remembers about the attack she got, how she felt about it, her fears of getting sick again. But Angela soon found herself writing about other aspects of her life as well. Somehow, Angela finds this journal deeply comforting. She couldn't say exactly why, but she has the sense that it is making her feel better.

Lydia is determined to get her life "back to normal." She wears a mask at work during the times of high exposure to flour in the air, and although her co-workers tease her about it at first, she just shrugs it off.

Lydia also decides that she has to make some other changes in her life. Because she's been feeling so sick and exhausted lately, she hasn't been able to keep up her normal schedule—and she's starting to realize that she didn't like that schedule so much anyway. She used to drive to her family's house for dinner every Sunday—a two-hour trip each way. When she got sick and couldn't make the drive so easily, she started to realize that she liked having Sundays as quiet time to herself. Lydia arranges with her family to visit twice a month instead of every week, which causes some conflicts at first, but she holds firmly to her resolution.

Lydia also realizes that she has let her boyfriend make all the plans for the two of them, with him choosing a lot of social time out at parties and bars. Because Lydia knows that she can't handle the smoky atmosphere any more, she feels braver about asking for a different kind of time together—more dinners with friends and quiet evenings at home together.

Lydia is still struggling with asthma—and she's still trying to decide whether she can keep the job that seems to be making her sick. But she's starting to feel good about some of the other changes she's making in her life.

## You and Your Body: A Holistic Approach

It's rare that a person with asthma goes to visit a doctor and says, "Basically, I feel great all the time—except when I have an asthma attack." Usually, asthma—like all diseases—is part of a bigger set of problems. That's because every part of the body affects every other part. If one part of your body is under stress, the rest of the body starts working overtime to help out, to compensate, or to counteract the problem. Thus, people with chronic asthma tend to suffer as well from fatigue, back pain, upper respiratory problems, headaches, and a general feeling of malaise.

Asthma is not a collection of symptoms to be treated as isolated instances. Rather, a *person* experiences asthma—among many other experiences. If you have asthma, everything that you do—everything you eat, every activity you engage in, every emotion you feel—affects your entire system, including your asthma. So looking at diet, exercise, breathing patterns, and the like becomes an integral part of regaining health. This chapter looks at factors affecting your emotions, your attitude, and your diet. The following chapter looks at general exercise and breathing exercises.

### *A Holistic Approach to* You

Many people, in order to figure out an approach to treatment, break things down: this for the body, that for the emotions. But remember that your body, your mind, and your emotions are really a single entity—they are *you.*

*The Emotional Side of Asthma*   An asthma attack is a physical experience—chest pain, coughing, difficulty breathing—but it is also an emotional experience—the anxiety of not being able to breathe, the frustration of not being able to do what you'd like to, the fear of when the next attack might come. Other emotions that people often feel around asthma (and other diseases) include shame (for being "out of control," "helpless," or "needy"), sadness, anger, triumph ("I *knew* there was something wrong with me! Now maybe you'll believe me!"), resentment ("Why is this happening to me?"), despair, loneliness, guilt ("I'm taking up too much of other people's time and attention" or "Other people need help so much more than I do."), and relief ("Now I don't have to [fill in the blank]," "Now it's finally my turn to be taken care of.").

*Asthma and Your Mind*  Asthma is also a mental experience. If you believe that your asthma is someone else's responsibility, that will lead to one way of dealing with it. If you believe that your asthma is *yours,* that you can explore and understand both your experience of sickness and your experience of health, that will lead you to other actions. What you think about your asthma, what you feel about it, and what you do about it, will all affect one another—and what you think, feel, and do will all affect your actual experience of the disease.

*Taking Responsibility*  Again, let's be very clear. If you have asthma, you are not "making yourself sick" or "choosing to be sick." Asthma is not primarily an emotional problem. You're getting it "on purpose," and you're getting it because you are thinking about it incorrectly.

*But* it's very helpful to look at yourself as a whole person whose mind, body, and emotions interact in profound and powerful ways. Sometimes a problem that begins in one area can be addressed in another. Even if a problem does not begin in your mind and emotions, sometimes your attitude or emotions can make an enormous difference in solving the problem. Suppose, for example, that one of your close friends was randomly hit by a car in a traffic accident. Clearly, the problem would have come from outside herself, not by her choice. Few people would claim that the problem began in either her mind or her emotions. Yet, once faced with the problem, your friend's attitude, her commitment to getting better, her feelings about herself and her body, and her general state of health would all make a tremendous difference in how fast and how fully she recovered from the accident.

*"The Home-Court Advantage"* Think of a top basketball team. The players know that a great deal of the game is physical. They depend on height, which they're born with; on talent, which they're born with but can also nurture; and on being in top physical shape, which has something to do with inheritance and even more to do with diet, exercise, and lifestyle. Moreover, good players know that if they visualize, say, making a free throw, they are far more likely to make the shot. Likewise, they know that if they go into a game "psyched" and ready to win, they can often overcome opponents that may be more powerful or more skilled, especially if those opponents are "psyched out" and discouraged.

The home-court advantage is the widely accepted belief that a team will play better when thousands of fans are cheering the players on. Do those cheering fans "make" the team win? Are they any substitute for practice, for eating right, for staying in shape, for simply having players who are tall and talented? If a team loses despite being on the home court, is it because they really "wanted" to lose, or because they somehow didn't "want to win *enough*"?

The answer to all those questions is a resounding NO. But successful athletes do understand the importance of morale, of emotional support, and of commitment to winning, just as "successful people with asthma" understand the importance of self-awareness, of emotional issues, and of commitment to health. No athlete wins every competition—and you may have some setbacks in your experience with asthma. But if you understand your mind and your body, and if you're committed to seeing yourself as a whole person, you can marshal all your resources—physical, emotional, and mental—behind your goal of health.

## Achieving Awareness

First, explore diet as an avenue to improved health, a more effective immune system, and a "less allergic" set of responses to your environment. (This is discussed at length later in this chapter.) Think of dietary changes in two ways: as a means to address your physical condition, and as a pathway to greater awareness. If you become more sensitive to the way your diet affects your mood, your energy, and your outlook, your experience of asthma and your ability to deal with asthma will be transformed.

To that end, begin with two more general suggestions about achieving awareness. These suggestions are *your* resources. If they appeal to you, work with them. If you have ideas for modifying them to better suit your needs, change them as you see fit. If you think they're not for you, skip them and read on about diet, exercise, and breathing. However, please remember that sometimes the suggestions that are the most meaningful also feel the most absurd or pointless, or provoke the most anxiety. So you might want to give at least one of the following ideas a chance:

### 1. Take Your Emotional Temperature

Take the following quiz. Try to respond as quickly as possible, following your first impulse. Take the quiz somewhere relatively private, with a notebook or a few blank pages handy, at a time when you have at least fifteen minutes of private, uninterrupted time. (If you can't imagine finding fifteen minutes of quiet time in your day, you might want to consider what that's telling you and whether you would enjoy having even a little more time to yourself!)

1. I feel nervous or uneasy much of the time. Yes ___ No ___
2. I feel that when I become too emotional—whether happy or sad—I might become short of breath. Yes ___ No ___
3. When I feel sad, there is no one to comfort me. Yes ___ No ___
4. When I feel confused or regretful, there is no one to help me figure out what to do. Yes ___ No ___
5. When I get angry, I have a hard time breathing. Yes ___ No ___
6. There really isn't much I can do to fix the things that bother me. Yes ___ No ___

7. Although some people care for me, I think that most people have either a negative or a neutral impression of me.  Yes ___ No ___

8. I think that if something makes you angry or upset, you should try to handle it alone, rather than impose it on someone else.  Yes ___ No ___

9. Getting help from others might be necessary sometimes, but it's better if people can handle problems by themselves.  Yes ___ No ___

10. I think that if someone really needs help, other people have a duty to do their best to help out.  Yes ___ No ___

Now, pick up your pen and the blank paper. Answer the following three questions, writing as much or as little as you like.

- Which of my answers surprises me the most?
- Which of my answers bothers me the most?
- How do I feel, now that I've thought about these issues?

There are no right or wrong answers to this quiz. It's simply a tool for finding out about your feelings, not a test to see if you have the "right" attitudes. However, if you answered yes to questions 1, 2, or 5, you may see your own emotions as potentially dangerous and likely to provoke an asthma attack. Working to become more comfortable with those emotions might help relieve your anxiety—and possibly, might also help relieve some asthma symptoms.

If you answered yes to questions 3, 4, or 7, you are probably feeling lonely and in need of emotional support. It might be helpful to think of people who could provide more support for you: a religious leader, a counselor or therapist, a trusted friend, a family member. You have a right to love, companionship, and guidance—you might want to take steps to get more of those qualities into your life.

If you answered yes to question 6, you might also consider how you might work with this attitude. Perhaps you need to focus on what you *can* do to change the things that bother you, even if you believe that what you can do is very limited. Perhaps you need to seek counseling, therapy, or religious support to expand your ideas of what's possible for you to achieve. Likewise, if you answer yes to question 9, you might consider trying to expand your thinking about this issue. It's very difficult to change—whether you're changing your diet, your habits of exercise, your mental outlook, or your health—without the help of other people. Feeling that it's better *not* to get help can handicap your efforts before you begin.

If you answered yes to question 8, you might consider whether "stuffing" your emotions is working for you. The stress of trying to handle everything alone, rather than sharing your feelings, may be putting you under an unnecessary strain.

Finally, if you answered yes to question 10, you might consider whether there are ways of getting comfort, support, and attention other than by being sick. Many people feel—even if they don't consciously agree with this feeling—that they can only get help from others when they are sick or needy. Otherwise, they feel that others' needs should come first. There may even be some reality to this feeling if you are a parent or you are responsible for aging family members. Nevertheless, *everyone* needs help, comfort, and support some of the time. If you have a chronic disease, such as asthma, it's important to know that you can get "babied" once in a while without being sick.

### 2. Keep an "Asthma Journal"

The advisability of keeping an asthma journal or a diary has already been mentioned several times. But instead of simply charting your symptoms, try going a step further. Allowing yourself twenty quiet minutes to write each day might be just the thing you need to reconnect with yourself. Some people like to write at the beginning of the day, some at the end, some when the spirit moves them. Some people prefer to give themselves a page quota—say, three pages a day; others prefer to pick a time limit, such as fifteen or twenty minutes. In either case, writing about your body, your memories, your feelings, your life experiences, can help you to know yourself better and can also provide a kind of grounding or centering, reminding you that you can always count on yourself.

The whole point of keeping a journal is to choose what you'd like to write about. But if you're looking for some suggestions, you might make use of these:

- My earliest asthma experience
- What it feels like to have an attack
- What I hate most about having asthma
- What I like most about having asthma
- How I feel about my family's treatment of me and my asthma
- Something that bothered me today
- Something that made me feel great today
- Some questions I have about myself, my health, my life
- A list of ten things I'd love to do–if only I could . . .
- If I were in perfect health, my idea of the perfect day

And, for the more ambitious:

- My asthma history–everything I remember about myself and my asthma, from my very first attack through the present (a work of several installments!)
- A day of asthma–how I feel about attacks that happen in the morning, in the afternoon, in the evening, at night (choose just one time of day for each day of writing)
- My life without asthma–my biography, or the life I would have had, if I had never had asthma (this might be one or more days' writing)

It's a certainty that if you keep a journal, whether you follow these suggestions or just let your writing flow where it will, you'll find out more about yourself–and you may even feel better!

## Eating for Health

What you breathe has an obvious impact on your asthma. What you eat has a less obvious but no less profound effect. As discussed earlier, eating allergens can keep inflammatory chemicals circulating in your body, making you more sensitive to a greater number of asthma triggers in the air and in your food. Some foods, such as fish oil, seem to reduce inflammation. A liver-friendly diet—low in fats, additives, preservatives, alcohol, and medications—can help your system cope with any stress. If you eat lots of sweets, or if you often crave sweets, you may have or may be giving yourself hypoglycemia (low blood sugar), whose symptoms of shakiness, panic, and weakness may be easily confused with asthma, creating a vicious cycle of anxiety and frustration over your health. And if you eat a healthy diet, perhaps supplemented with certain vitamins and minerals, you may support your body's immune system and increase your ability to avoid or withstand asthma attacks.

Let's start with another quiz. The answers could help you determine some vitamin and mineral deficiencies that you might remedy through better nutrition and/or taking supplements. CAUTION: *Do not follow these recommendations on your own.* Work with a doctor or nutritionist who understands not only the effects of various vitamins and minerals but also how different supplements interact with one another, with any medications you may be taking, and with your body as a whole.

### *Do I Suffer from Vitamin or Mineral Deficiency?*

1. I have dry, rough skin, dry eyes, and/or night blindness.  Yes ___ No ___

2. I bruise easily, my wounds heal slowly, my gums bleed easily, I have nosebleeds, and/or I get frequent infections.  Yes ___ No ___

3. I often experience one or more of the following: headaches, nausea, vomiting,

     depression, fatigue, constipation,
     irritability, lack of appetite.     Yes ___ No ___

4. My tongue is often inflamed, I have cracks at the corners of my mouth, or I have patches of dry, itchy skin.     Yes ___ No ___

5. I often feel weak, my tongue is sore, I have back pains, or I lose weight more easily than I would like.     Yes ___ No ___

6. I frequently get headaches, have trouble sleeping, feel anemic, feel weak, or feel irritable.     Yes ___ No ___

7. I feel that my muscles are weaker than they should be; I'm often extremely tired; sometimes I get dizzy; or sometimes I feel tingling in my fingers and toes.     Yes ___ No ___

8. My hair is dull, my skin is lackluster, I don't taste my food very well, I have a poor appetite, and/or my wounds heal very slowly.     Yes ___ No ___

9. I often get muscle cramps and spasms, feel tired, feel tense and irritable, or suffer from poor coordination.     Yes ___ No ___

If you answered yes to a particular question, you may be suffering from any one of a number of diseases (Addison's, thyroid, cancer) or from a shortage of the following vitamins or minerals:

    1. vitamin A     4. vitamin $B_6$     7. iron
    2. vitamin C     5. vitamin $B_{12}$     8. zinc
    3. vitamin $B_1$     6. folic acid     9. magnesium

Again, *work with your doctor or nutritionist* in identifying and addressing any possible deficiencies or other disorders causing these symptoms.

## Nutritional Principles

As you've probably gathered by now, you and your own sense of your health are your own best guide to what diet is best for you. Your next best resource is a doctor or nutritionist who can help you identify your particular needs. To supplement those two resources, here are some general recommendations for diet:

- A low-fat diet will help you maintain normal weight. Avoid or cut down on red meat, fried foods, butter/margarine, and fatty desserts.
- Do eat lots of whole grains, fresh fruits and vegetables, sea vegetables (high in calcium, a good dairy substitute!), and fish.
- Get to know the foods that you are allergic to (see the section on elimination diets in Chapter 5) and avoid or cut down on them. In conjunction with your physician, figure out which foods you need to cut out.
- Be aware of the most common food allergens: wheat, dairy, soy, eggs, seeds.

## Helpful Nutrients

Many people believe that it is helpful to supplement their diets with extra vitamins and minerals. Again, *make these dietary changes only with the help of a doctor or nutritionist.* You may respond well to some of the following nutrients; but there may be some to which your particular system will respond badly. Here is a brief list of some supplements and their recommended doses.

- *Vitamin E* is an antioxidant that combats the damaging effects of ozone and smog. (400 IU [international units] a day)
- *Vitamin C* is an antioxidant that stimulates white blood cells to fight infection, and helps prevent cataracts. (up to 1 gram per day)
- *Beta-carotene* fights the aging process, is possibly associated with the ability to fight lung cancer, and converts to vitamin A. (25,000 IU a day)

- *B vitamins*, especially $B_5$, $B_6$, and $B_{12}$, may help combat fatigue, boost the immune system, and may help combat asthma. (50 mg of $B_2$ and $B_3$; 100 mg of $B_1$; 500 mg of $B_5$; 150 mg of $B_6$; 1,000 micrograms of $B_{12}$)
- *Zinc* promotes healing. (25 mg a day) (CAUTION: Excess levels of zinc can displace other minerals and may be linked to health problems.)
- *Vitamin A* supports the epithelium, the tissue that lines the airways, mouth, and nose. (5,000 IU a day) (CAUTION: Excess vitamin A can be toxic!)
- *Selenium* protects cell membranes and protects against toxins. (200 micrograms a day)

Two of the most popular but unproven herbal supplements are ginseng (400 mg twice a day) and Echinacea (400 mg twice a day).

Remember that the placebo effect yields benefits in 40 to 50 percent of disorders, so that complicates the evaluation of supplements unless double-blind placebo controlled studies are done.

Although research into the relationship of nutrition and asthma is still incomplete, some results suggest that certain supplements may be particularly helpful to people with asthma. Once again, *work with a doctor or nutritionist* to find the nutritional supplements that are right for you. Some supplements you might consider include the following:

- *Magnesium*: The muscles around the bronchial tubes constrict in part because there is an imbalance of calcium and magnesium there. It's a delicate balance: either too much or too little calcium can produce a muscle spasm; without calcium, the muscles can't move at all. Magnesium seems to displace excess calcium in cells and so may be helpful for people with asthma. Magnesium also seems to make asthma patients' lungs less "twitchy" and more able to expel air. Studies have shown that during an asthma attack, blood levels of magnesium are down, while histamine levels are up. For these reasons, consider taking magnesium supplements under the supervision of a health care professional.

- *Omega-3 fatty acids:* These "natural lubricants," found in fish oils, are absorbed right into your cells. They seem to help cells reverse inflammation naturally. It may take ten weeks or more for fish oil to have any effect. (CAUTION: Fish oils contain vitamin A, which can be toxic in high quantities, so *do not self-medicate* with vitamins and fish oil supplements; work with a nutritionist.)

It cannot be stressed too often that these are all potent substances that can have powerful effects either alone or in combination with other nutrients, supplements, and medications. DO NOT TREAT YOURSELF BY YOURSELF. Make sure that whomever you work with is aware of EVERY medication, supplement, and vitamin that you are taking. Remember that the FDA does not control content or declare the safety of any food supplements.

### Gastrointestinal Reflux

This intestinal problem may be linked to asthma attacks. Normally, two sphincter muscles guard each entrance to the stomach, to make sure that no food leaves the stomach until it has been properly digested. The cardiac sphincter relaxes to let food into the stomach and then contracts to keep food there. The pyloric sphincter contracts the passage that leads to the intestines.

If you have indigestion, however, you may experience gastrointestinal reflux, in which the cardiac sphincter relaxes enough to allow food to leak back up into the esophagus. You may experience this as burping, belching, or feeling food actually rise back up into your throat. One theory is that the acidity and the undigested food is actually aspirated into the lungs and triggers an asthma attack. Another theory is that acid irritates the vagus nerve in the esophagus, which is a branch of the parasympathetic nervous system. Somehow, the vagus nerve, which serves both the stomach and the lungs, translates the irritation of indigestion into an asthma attack.

As you can see, we don't understand exactly how "GI reflux" and asthma are connected—but they do seem to be linked. If you suffer frequently from indigestion, you may wish to explore dietary changes, both to decrease the reflux and perhaps to calm your asthma.

*Preventing GI Reflux Attacks*  To prevent nighttime GI reflux attacks, elevate the head of your bed by 4 to 6 inches; eat smaller, more frequent meals; avoid food or drink near bedtime; and avoid fatty or spicy foods, alcohol, caffeine, and the medication theophylline. (Of course, if your doctor has prescribed theophylline for you, talk to him or her before discontinuing it.) Remember that chocolate and peppermint also contain caffeine-like substances and should be avoided.

### Making Changes

As shown throughout this book, it can feel overwhelming to make changes in any part of your life. Becoming more aware of the connection between mind and body, changing your diet, and developing new approaches to your asthma can be profoundly unsettling—as well as deeply rewarding.

The best approach is to take it one day at a time. If wholesale changes seem overwhelming, start with one little change. Build in a five-minute break in the midst of a busy workday, cut out one potential asthma trigger from your diet, or commit to writing one journal page per day. Once you've gotten comfortable with one change, consider making another. You may be surprised at how quickly you get used to your new habits.

### Ask Your Doctor . . .

- How can we work together to identify the changes I might need to make in my life, my lifestyle, my diet, and my exercise habits? What would you like to know? What areas should I focus on?
- How is my nutrition?
- What are the best foods for me?
- What are the allergenic foods for me?
- What are generally healthy foods for me?

- What foods should I avoid?
- Am I suffering from shortages–possibly even subclinical shortages–of some essential nutrient?
- Do I need vitamin or mineral supplements?
- Would magnesium supplements help me?
- How about omega-3 fatty acids?
- Are there other herbs or extracts that might help my condition?
- Do you know about specific research into nutrition or other areas that might relate to my condition?

# 9

# Breathing Well: Exercise Your Lungs

Malcolm is so excited about the way that changing his diet has improved his health and spirits that he starts making other changes in his life. He realizes that he needs to find a form of exercise that will work for him—something that won't set off an asthma attack but that will still give his lungs a vigorous workout.

Malcolm consults with his doctor to find a kind of exercise that he can do safely and comfortably. After exploring a number of options, he finally settles on working out with weights. (CAUTION: This may not be the best exercise for someone with gastrointestinal reflux.) The doctor advises him to stretch before doing any vigorous activity, to keep his inhaler handy, and to stay aware and "in touch" with his body. After a few weeks of weight training, Malcolm notices that he is calmer, more relaxed, and generally in a better mood. He is also sleeping better and noticing fewer asthma symptoms.

Angela's doctor starts treating her for asthma. But he tells her that he doesn't just want to give her medication—he also wants her to restore her system to health. He and Angela work out an exercise plan, in which Angela takes a vigorous walk three times a week and goes swimming at the local "Y" three times a week. The doctor tells Angela to make sure to do stretches and warm-ups before she exercises, and he explains how she can avoid "exercise-induced asthma." Within a few weeks, Angela notices that she is breathing more deeply and more easily, and that she has lost that sense of perennial exhaustion.

So Angela starts exploring a few more changes. She goes to a yoga class, where she learns some breathing exercises that she practices all the time. The yoga teacher even shows her some exercises she can do during an attack or when she feels an attack coming on. Angela feels better just knowing that there is something she can do besides taking medication.

## Why Exercise?

There are so many good reasons to exercise, it's hard to know where to start. Your body was designed to move, to use itself, even to push itself to some extent. Using your muscles and your energy will, paradoxically, make you stronger and give you more energy. Aerobic exercise—exercise that depends on deep, vigorous breathing—is clearly good for everyone's lungs, and it is of especially important benefit if you have asthma. Moreover, excess weight can complicate asthma, and exercise can help you lose weight.

There is also some evidence that exercise is good for the immune system. Some studies have shown that the "suppressor reaction"—the one that orders inflammatory chemicals in your body to subside—is strengthened during exercise. Although the count of suppressor T-cells apparently rises during exercise and falls again afterward, exercise may still be a chance for your body to "calm down" from its heightened state of allergic overreaction.

Finally, some forms of exercise, notably yoga and t'ai chi, involve deep breathing, mental relaxation, and a meditative use of mind and body together. People who practice these forms of exercise report not only dramatic physical benefits—stronger bodies, more energy, greater flexibility, weight loss—but also enormous mental and emotional benefits, including a sense of calm, an openness to new ideas, a friendlier relationship with their bodies and their world.

*Exercise and Awareness* As with diet, exercise has a double function. Just being involved in physical activity is likely to boost your general level of health. But in addition, exercise can help you achieve a greater level of body awareness—awareness that can pay off in your treatment of asthma. If exercise helps you experience what your body is capable of, what it needs and wants; if you get in touch with your breathing and learn to work with it rather than losing touch with it during an asthma attack—your experience of asthma and its symptoms is also likely to change.

## Making Exercise Safe

Body awareness is the key to making exercise safe and healthy. You might have heard the slogan "No pain, no gain"; you may even know coaches or athletes who promote this philosophy. But it's important to realize that there are two types of pain: The type that brings gain is the muscle burn that you feel during a vigorous workout. The type that can actually set your health back is the pain that comes from your body trying to tell you that you're doing too much. If you feel a shooting pain or tearing sensation in any muscle, for example, *stop immediately;* you may have torn a ligament. And if you're suffering from a respiratory infection or from asthma, and you try to "push your body through the pain," you can end up making yourself sicker.

Olympic champion swimmer Nancy Hogshead has asthma. With Gerald S. Couzens, she wrote *Asthma and Exercise,* a book that recounts her own experience and gives advice to others with asthma. Hogshead cautions:

> I stop swim workouts immediately whenever I feel the first twinge of pain in my shoulder or feel that I've reached a point where my asthma is coming on. In times of pain like this, it doesn't help you become a better athlete if you continue to push your body through a workout. Whatever is bothering you will only get worse if you continue to exercise, and could set your training back for an indefinite period.
>
> It always pays to be aware of your asthma status. If you feel your asthma is particularly aggravated by colds and flus, then ease up a bit on your exercise program if you have the sniffles, body aches, or feel particularly run-down. You might even con-

sider eliminating a workout or two until you feel completely better. There is nothing wimpish about this. A world-class athlete pushes his or her body in one sense, but knows how to baby it as well.

## *Pollution and Exercise*

If you're planning to exercise outdoors, you need to be aware of air pollution. As a general principle, the benefits your lungs and body derive from exercising—say, jogging, walking briskly, or playing tennis—are far greater than the dangers of breathing in air pollutants. However, on some days and in some cases, the amount of pollution you're exposed to may tip the scale. Although you may get used to the initial effects of breathing in ozone, you won't escape its long-term—and irreversible—damage to your lungs.

If you live in a city or in an area with lots of traffic, try to do outdoor exercise in the morning, before 10 A.M., when the air is cleaner, rather than in the afternoon. Avoid jogging or walking on busy streets if you possibly can. Once ozone levels are high, they generally remain so until early evening.

You can use this chart to determine which days are safe for you to exercise outdoors. It's based on the Pollution Standard Index (PSI), which takes into account both the regional ozone level and several other air-pollution factors. This figure should be available from the regional office of your state Department of Environmental Conservation.

### Pollution Standard Index

| | | |
|---:|:---:|:---|
| 0–49 | = | Good* |
| 50–99 | = | Moderate* |
| 100–199 | = | Unhealthful |
| 200–299 | = | Very unhealthful |
| 300–500 | = | Hazardous |

\* safe to exercise

## *Avoiding Exercise-Induced Asthma (EIA)*

Some 60 to 90 percent of those who have asthma sometimes respond to exercise as an asthma trigger. If you have asthma and you perform an athletic activity—running, skiing, swimming, cycling, basketball, aerobics—for five minutes or more at 70 percent of your aerobic (lung) capacity, you can trigger an asthma attack. However, exercise-induced asthma is reversible. You just have to take some care—and, once again, be aware.

EIA (also known as exercise-induced bronchospasm [EIB]) seems to be caused by cool, dry air passing into the lungs as the exerciser breathes more rapidly, so that the nose and mouth have less of a chance to warm and humidify the inhaled air. Its symptoms include shortness of breath; coughing; wheezing; a tight, burning feeling in the chest; abdominal pain; headache; and fatigue. If you weren't having an asthma attack before you began to exercise, these symptoms will usually clear up by themselves. Otherwise, an inhaler with a bronchodilator will expand the airways and stop an episode fairly soon. Some athletes recommend either taking a few puffs of an inhaler (check with your physician as to which medication to use) about twenty to thirty minutes before starting to exercise or taking oral medication an hour before exercise. Other athletes have been able to manage their EIA without medication, using some of these suggestions:

- *Avoid cold, dry air if possible—or wear a mask.* You can get special masks with air filters in them for jogging, brisk walking, or skiing outdoors in winter. If you take up swimming, you'll be breathing the perfectly conditioned warm, humid air from just above the surface of a heated pool. However, some swimmers react to mold and/or chlorine.
- *Breathe through the nose rather than the mouth.* The nose was designed to filter, warm, and humidify the air we breathe.
- *Warm up gradually.* EIA symptoms usually start about five minutes after you've reached your peak exercise exertion. If you can "run through" your symptoms by starting out slowly and exercising at a low level until symptoms subside, you are then usually free to work yourself up to your peak.
- *Cool down after you've reached your peak.*

## Recommended Warm-Up and Cool-Down Schedules to Avoid EIA without Medication

### Schedule #1

*Before Exercise*

Two- to three-minute warm-up exercises, alternating with rest periods; for up to forty minutes.

*During Exercise*

Breathe warm, humid air, through your nose, for less than five minutes of maximum exertion. If you like, you can repeat five minutes of peak exercise exertion after another forty minutes of warm-up.

*After Exercise*

Take deep, slow breaths.

However, many people with asthma simply prefer to take medication before exercise. In that case, you might eventually work your way up to a schedule like the following:

### Schedule #2

*Before Exercise*

Ten to twenty minutes of stretching

Five minutes of warm-up

*During Exercise*

Fifteen to sixty minutes of aerobic exercise

*After Exercise*

Five minutes of cool-down

Five minutes of stretching

## Recommended Exercise

The best exercise for you is probably the exercise that you enjoy the most. You might want to experiment with different types of exercise or work out an exercise program that includes a variety of activities. Experiment and enjoy yourself. Of course, as with all things, consult your doctor before beginning, and stay in close touch with him or her if you experience any problems.

*Aerobic Exercise* Your exercise should include at least some aerobic exercise, however, unless you do yoga or t'ai chi, which will strengthen your lungs and improve your breathing in a different way. Aerobic exercise includes walking, race walking, jogging, swimming, cycling, cross-country skiing, rowing, canoeing, roller skating, climbing stairs, dancing, jumping rope, step routines, aerobics classes, hiking, tennis, racquetball, and squash.

*Warm-Ups and Cool-Downs* If you do engage in aerobic exercise, make sure that you stretch before and after exercise. Stretching is one of those invisible activities, like housework, that you don't always notice when you do it—but that sooner or later catches up with you when you don't do it. Consider that stretching is not only good for your muscles: it also promotes relaxation, seems to have some antiaging benefits, and helps you be more flexible mentally as well as physically.

## Breathing

As discussed earlier, the primary purpose of breathing is to extract oxygen from the atmosphere and make it available to the body's cells. However, breathing also serves an important psychological function: it's very calming. Naturally, we feel anxious when we have difficulty breathing. In addition, feeling anxious makes it hard to breathe, causing breaths to come more rapidly and shallowly. But breathing deeply and slowly can actually help to soothe anxious feelings. Actors and singers have long known the value of deep breathing as an antidote to stage fright, for example.

*Hyperventilation* When you breathe rapidly, in the shallow, rapid breathing typical of the anxious "fight-or-flight" reaction triggered by an adrenaline rush of anxiety, you are actually hyperventilating—and decreasing carbon dioxide, leading to electrolyte shifts that can make you feel dizzy, faint, disoriented, and panicked.

### Breathing Exercises

People with asthma can benefit enormously from doing regular breathing exercises, both as a daily practice and as a way to respond to an asthma attack. If you can synchronize your breathing and your heart rate, you can get into a meditative state, which again, is very calming, whether you enter it during an attack or as a regular activity. Moreover, most people have about 20 percent "extra" lung capacity that they don't normally use. Regular breathing exercises can help bring that 20 percent into use–an advantage of enormous benefit to people with asthma, who work harder than normal to breathe during an attack.

*Biofeedback* You may wish to explore biofeedback with a psychologist as a way to improve your breathing. A sophisticated machine monitors your breathing and feeds back information to you through sound and light signals. You lie quietly on your back while an infrared sensor on your upper abdomen responds to your breathing. A headset over your eyes and ears blocks out outside noise and light. Meanwhile, you receive gentle sound and light cues to help you realize when you are not breathing properly, from your diaphragm. Most people learn to breathe properly, to achieve deep relaxation, within four thirty-minute sessions.

You can also buy a machine called the Breathwork Explorer, which helps you learn to breathe from the diaphragm. It costs about $350.

### Teach Yourself to Breathe

However, you can teach yourself correct breathing, without help from a machine. Then you simply need to remember to practice!

*Breathing Deeply* Proper breathing is both easier and harder than it sounds. On the one hand, our bodies are constructed to breathe "properly"–that is, deeply, gently, and from the diaphragm. Over time, however, we acquire numerous bad habits for all sorts of physical and psychological reasons. At this point, learning to breathe properly is mainly a matter of undoing bad habits.

Look at yourself in the mirror. Breathe in. Can you see your shoulders lift? If so, your first step is to learn to relax your shoulders. Does your chest stiffen as well? Those are extra muscles that you don't need for breathing—and if you use those muscles during an asthma attack, you'll tire yourself out that much more quickly.

Now, feel where the air goes. Place your hand lightly on your abdomen, just below the navel. If you are breathing deeply and properly, you will feel your stomach push out gently as you breathe in, returning to a flatter position as you breathe out. (Many people have reversed this natural pattern, sucking their stomachs in as they inhale, and puffing them out as they exhale. This creates tension and deprives you of oxygen.) You should feel each breath go all the way down into your diaphragm (the area below your rib cage). Shallow breathing, which stays in your upper lungs, does not relax you and it provides you with less oxygen.

Next, count your breaths. How many times per minute do you breathe? More than fourteen, and your breathing is probably too rapid and shallow. Normal breathing is about twelve times a minute; deep, diaphragmatic breathing can be as slow as three or four breaths per minute.

### *Calm Yourself Through Breathing*

Here is one simple exercise that can help you relax, calm down, and breathe deeply. This exercise is excellent for times when you feel yourself becoming tense, such as when you're caught in a traffic jam, when you're meeting a work deadline, or when you're becoming increasingly anxious or frustrated in any situation.

- Breathe in on a count of one, and breathe out on a count of one.
- Breathe in on a count of two, and breathe out on a count of two.
- Breathe in on a count of three, and breathe out on a count of three.
- Continue until you are breathing in on a count of twelve, and out on a count of twelve.

Be careful not to hold your breath to make the count. Avoid pushing or straining. Visualize your lungs and diaphragm as gently opening to receive more and more air. Feel each breath travel down through your lungs and into your diaphragm. Feel how your entire body expands and relaxes as you receive this precious air. Focus on the feeling of the breath, and on keeping your count even and steady.

Since the entire exercise can be completed in less than three minutes (although you're certainly free to continue breathing slowly, on a count of ten, twelve, or whatever is comfortable for you, for as long as you like), you can easily rationalize taking a short "breathing" break, even in the midst of a deadline. Remind yourself that this exercise gets more oxygen to your brain and will therefore refresh you, make your mind sharper, and make you far more efficient when you resume work.

## *Breathing Exercises to Relax and Energize You*

Here is a comprehensive program of breathing exercises. After only a few days, you should notice a renewed sense of relaxation and energy. Over a few months, you'll find that you've greatly expanded your breathing capacity.

NOTE: If you ever feel light-headed during these exercises, stop a moment and breathe as you normally would.

### 1. Use your diaphragm: the basics

- Lie on your back on the floor, using a mat or blanket if necessary. (No pillows, though—you want your back and neck to be entirely flat.) Raise your knees, keeping your feet flat on the floor and your legs slightly apart.
- Put a hardcover book on your stomach (just below your navel), with the binding just touching the bottom of your rib cage.
- Breathe in, through your nose if at all possible. Visualize, though, that you are drawing the air from the back of your throat. The air will feel as though it were coming from inside you.
- As you inhale, try to lift the book as high as you can, while keeping your chest flat and still. If necessary, put one hand gently on your chest, to remind it not to move.

- Visualize your stomach as a balloon that you are gradually, gently filling with oxygen. (Your chest will also expand slightly, toward the end of the breath.) Some people like to mentally repeat the expression, "The breath falls in," and then, when they exhale, "The breath falls out."

- When you exhale, use the same muscles that lifted the book to squeeze every last drop of air out of your body. It should take you longer to exhale than to inhale. If you need to slow yourself down, try inhaling on a slow count of four and exhaling on a slow count of first six, then eight.

- When you have almost finished exhaling, hum. You may be surprised at how much breath you have left! Keep humming until you are out of air.

- Ideally, you would take only four breaths per minute with this exercise. After you've practiced it for a while, you might try timing yourself.

**2. Use your diaphragm: three variations**

- Again, lie on the floor, on your back with your knees raised and your feet about 8 inches apart on the floor. Rock gently on your coccyx, or tailbone—the bone at the base of the spine. (You may wish to lie on a blanket or exercise mat.) Arch your back slightly as you inhale; roll your back onto the floor as you exhale.

- Lie on your back as before. Swing your knees to your chest as you inhale. Lower them back to their original position as you exhale.

- Sit upright in a comfortable, straight chair. Relax your entire body. (Some people like to imagine that they are releasing all their tension as they exhale. They visualize the tension slipping away, from the crown of the head down through the neck, chest, arms, stomach, legs, and feet.) Put each hand palm down against either side, with your fingers under your ribs and your thumbs against your back. As you inhale, you should feel your hands move forward; as you exhale, you'll feel them move back. This is a good position in which to slow your breathing by progressively increasing the count, as in Exercise 1.

### 3. Blow out the candle

- Choose any position: sitting, standing, or lying down.
- Draw in a deep breath.
- When you exhale, purse your lips and blow hard, as if you were blowing out a candle.

### 4. Shoulder drop

This is an excellent exercise for learning to relax your shoulders while breathing.

- Stand with your feet about 12 inches apart, your arms dangling.
- Bend your head forward, stretching the back of your neck.
- Inhale deeply, feeling your stomach expand.
- Swing your arms to the right, then to the left, while inhaling.
- Exhale deeply.
- Inhale again.
- Exhale a second time, vigorously, through pursed lips. While exhaling, lower your shoulders as you slowly bring your head up. Gently tilt your head back. (Be careful not to overextend your neck.) As your head falls back, on the exhale, swing your arms to the left and then to the right.
- On your next inhale, once again, let your head fall forward.
- On your next exhale, with your head forward, swing your arms to the right and left.

### 5. Chest stretch

This exercise will help open and relax your chest, lungs, and diaphragm.

- Stand straight, with your feet about shoulder width.
- Lower your shoulders—and relax them! Shake your arms, to make sure your upper body is relaxed, letting your hands dangle at your sides.
- Inhale.
- Exhale while stretching your head back as far as possible, being careful not to overextend the neck.
- Inhale again, while straightening up.
- Repeat several times.

### 6. Breathe into your feelings

This is an excellent exercise that will help you use breathing to relax. Whenever you feel something strongly—panic, fear, anger, anxiety, frustration, resentment—you are likely to go into fight-or-flight shallow breathing. Likewise, whenever an asthma attack begins, your system will tend to respond with panic and alarm—and rapid, shallow breathing.

When this happens, remind yourself to breathe *into* the feelings. This is where all that body awareness comes in handy! Notice which parts of your body are tense—your jaw, scalp, hands, feet, face, chest, neck, back? Breathe into the part of the body that is tense, imagining a soft, loving breath helping the tense area to expand on the inhale, relax on the exhale.

Allow yourself to breathe *with* the feelings. You may find yourself laughing, crying, or reacting in some other vocal way. Allow your reactions to happen as you continue to focus on breathing deeply and gently. You may feel the impulse to cut your feelings short with shallow breathing or tense muscles. Focus on your breathing. Breathe deeply, all the way into the diaphragm. If necessary, use a count to help you slow your breathing down.

You may find that this exercise helps mitigate, interrupt, or even end an asthma attack. However, don't forget to use your medications as instructed by your physician. If the attack is severe, call your physician or go to the emergency room of your hospital.

### 7. The bellows

You may need some time to work up to this exercise. But just one round of this vigorous exercise will help relax you. Repeated rounds will help strengthen your diaphragm muscles and expand your breathing capacity.

- Sit in a chair and breathe deeply.
- As you exhale, lean forward from the waist, slowly, as you pull your diaphragm muscles in, so that by the end of your exhalation, your head is close to your knees.
- Purse your lips and hiss as you pull your diaphragm in further and expel the last bit of air in your lungs.
- As you breathe in, slowly raise yourself to a sitting position, so that by the time you have finished breathing in deeply, you are sitting upright.
- Then exhale quickly and lean forward quickly, as though you've been punched. Suck in your diaphragm, purse your lips, and force the air out powerfully. As your exhale finishes, hiss.
- Relax, breathe in, and sit up slowly once more.

### 8. Breathe with your heart

The object of this exercise is to coordinate your breathing and your heartbeat. It can help you achieve a meditative state and is a wonderfully calming response to an asthma attack.

- Put one hand on your stomach, with two fingers of the other hand on the first hand's pulse.
- Synchronize your breathing and your heart: for every seven heartbeats, breathe in. For every nine heartbeats, breathe out.

*Ask Your Doctor . . .*

- What kind of exercise regime do you recommend for me?
- What precautions should I take regarding exercise?
- Can you help me—or can you recommend someone to help me—learn to breathe properly?
- What other parts of the mind-body connection should I be attending to?

# 10

# Alternative Strategies for Treating Asthma

Malcolm decides that in addition to working with a nutritionist, he would like to explore herbal medicine. He's read that Siberian ginseng, mullein, fenugreek, catnip, sage, passion flower, eucalyptus, and angelica can all help relieve asthma symptoms and calm people's allergies. Malcolm goes to the local health-food store, and he finds many of these herbs on the shelves–but in so many different combinations and brand names that he feels totally overwhelmed. Part of him is sure that it doesn't matter, that these weird preparations can't possibly help him or hurt him, because after all, they're not medicine. They're just herbs. But another part of him believes that if he takes the wrong thing, he could make himself even sicker.

Malcolm discovers that many people practice herbal medicine to treat a wide variety of diseases, including asthma. Some of these herbalists also practice acupuncture or have a background in Chinese medicine. Others follow the ayurvedic tradition of India. Still others are North American herbalists, who specialize in "local" herbs and do not necessarily practice the Chinese tradition. Malcolm feels more overwhelmed than he did before. How will he ever choose?

Angela decides that she wants to supplement her medical care with acupuncture. She's heard that people use acupuncture to help them relax and to treat headaches and stress-related illnesses. She wonders if an acupuncturist could also treat her asthma—and if so, whether that would free her from medication? But Angela knows that acupuncture involves needles of some kind—and needles make her nervous. She's not sure what to do.

When Lydia is looking into occupational asthma, she meets another woman with asthma who tells her that self-hypnosis can be extremely effective. This woman says that she made herself a tape, which she listens to periodically, especially when she feels she is in danger of an attack. Listening to the tape has also enabled her to go into a trance whenever she feels an attack coming on, even if there's no tape player available. Lydia doesn't understand the explanation very well, but it seems that somehow, the trance helps this woman avoid the attack. Lydia is intrigued—but also uncertain. How can she find out more?

## Exploring Alternative Strategies

Dr. Renata Engler, Chief of Allergy-Immunology at the Walter Reed Army Medical Center, has compiled extensive data on alternative systems of medical practice. In *Alternative Medicine Expanding Medical Horizons,* a paper she delivered to the National Institutes of Health, she reported that only ten to thirty percent of health care around the world is delivered by the biomedical practitioners we conventionally think of as healthcare providers. She believes that patients turn to alternative care because they do not feel that their physicians listen to them, because they want to be in control of their own treatments, and because at times they look for easy solutions to their problems. People tend to think that "natural" substances are better and safer than artificially produced material, and they often forget that some naturally occurring substances—for example, some mushrooms—can be highly toxic.

Many remedies are marketed as immune enhancers, and effective therapies for allergies and asthma. Some of these remedies have a long history of use, but information about their benefits beyond their placebo effect is limited. Expensive studies would have to be done to prove their efficacy and safety, but pharmaceutical companies cannot patent these natural substances and so are unlikely to fund such testing. Of course, many drugs are derived from plant sources. The new Office for Alternative Medical Research has been established at the NIH, but funding for these controlled studies remains limited. The FDA issues warnings occasionally, after deaths or serious injuries have been linked to these substances (for example, studies were done on the connection between chaparral and severe liver damage), but there is no official reporting mechanism that can be used to collect data. Many herbs that have been linked to serious injuries are still widely available, and their sales are not restricted.

The placebo effect is very real. Something happens in the body when patients expect to be helped. This is why every scientific study of a new drug or treatment includes a group of patients given placebos, so they can be compared with the group receiving the active substance under review. Dr. Engler suggests that this effect should be called "remembered wellness," which has positive connotations. However, this effect makes it difficult for individual patients to know whether their symptoms improve because they expect them to, or because of the substances they are taking.

## Herbal Medicine: What Is Known about the Efficacy and Safety of Herbs?

Echinacea (purple coneflower) has been studied extensively, but researchers have found no reported adverse side effects except for rare allergic reactions. It has been classified as a nonspecific stimulant of the immune system.

Herbs that have been associated with death or serious injury include artemisia (wormwood), belladonna, black cohosh, chamomile, chaparral, coltsfoot, comfrey root, kombuchea tea, lobelia, ma huang (ephedra), pennyroyal, sassafras, senna, and yohimbe, according to an article the *Washington Post* published on March 25, 1996.

Dr. Engler says that "There is an urgent need for further research to explore differences between suppliers and potential dosing or formulation differences.... Particularly for herbal remedies, there are no requirements for standardization of content so that different manufacturers may vary widely in actual active ingredient content." She warns her patients, "It is important to remember that use of complementary medicine constitutes a type of self-experimentation and carries unknown risk for the individual."

## Acupuncture

The basic theory of acupuncture is the notion of *chi,* an electromagnetic life force that flows through the blood, directed by the mind, giving energy and "spirit." The pathways through which *chi* flows are known as meridians, which conduct energy throughout the body, to organs and tissues. In Asian medicine, then, illness includes such conditions as exhaustion, indigestion, menstrual problems, and other "minor" issues, as well as the "clinical" illnesses of Western medicine, because any departure from perfect health and energy is viewed as a problem of *chi.*

More specifically, illnesses are seen as resulting from an imbalance or blockage of a person's *chi.* Acupuncture is the art of using tiny needles, the size of fine wire or thread, to stimulate various meridians to help restore the flow of *chi* and rebalance the body's energy. People who have experienced acupuncture often report feeling very relaxed very quickly; it's common for people to fall asleep during acupuncture treatments. This relaxation reflects the rebalancing of vital energy.

*What an Acupuncturist Will Do* Note that some physicians are also licensed to provide this care, and only they are recommended. Specifically, in a treatment, the acupuncturist will insert several needles, from one-half inch to one inch apart, in various parts of the body, most commonly the ears, the stomach, the face, and the feet, as well as along the extremities. Sometimes needles are inserted and removed immediately. Other times, they are left in for up to forty-five minutes. Techniques and placement vary.

Although the notion of "inserting needles" sounds painful and traumatic, it actually involves virtually no discomfort, although sometimes there is a slight pricking sensation just at the moment that the needle is inserted. Once the needle is in, however, the person being treated is rarely aware of it, and as mentioned, often feels relaxed and even falls asleep. Most acupuncturists will leave patients alone during the treatment, perhaps with a tape of soothing music playing in the background.

*The Limits of Acupuncture* Finally, remember that no treatment plan should offer to cure asthma. The most you can expect is a reduction of symptoms—and if you are seeing a physician who does acupuncture, you will probably need to invest at least six to ten weeks before seeing any results.

## Osteopathy

Osteopaths complete rigorous education equivalent to M.D.s and occupy the ground between alternative, holistic healing and Western medical science, with a great deal of overlap from both. The name "osteopath" comes from the Greek word *os*, which means "bone." Osteopathy is literally the study of how your bones fit together. More generally, osteopaths are interested in your posture and gait, and in the way that various parts of your body might block or restrict movement. Skin changes, reflex activity, and other signs of physical distress also provide important clues to osteopaths looking to get a sense of your physical system as a whole.

*Your First Visit* An initial visit to an osteopath should include a thorough evaluation and whatever tests he or she deems necessary. These will go hand in hand with questions about your environment, lifestyle, exercise habits, emotional life, and nutrition. If allergies seem to be a factor in your asthma, you may have to be referred for an allergy evaluation. (See Chapters 2 and 5 for more information about tests.)

After the osteopath has examined you, he or she will probably ask you to address several areas of your physical health: nutrition, vitamin and mineral supplements, or other alternative therapies. The goal of the osteopath is to come up with a highly individualized program that is suited to your specific physical condition.

## Chiropractic

The basic principle of chiropractic medicine is the relationship of the spinal column and the body's musculoskeletal structures to the nervous system. Every one of the body's organs, including the lungs, is linked to the spinal cord by a series of nerves. Therefore, chiropractors believe that when an organ is in distress, the reaction of the nerves causes the vertebrae to misalign. By the same token, if the body is misaligned, it causes distress to the various nerves, which in turn transmit the distress to "their" organs.

Therefore, chiropractors believe that by manipulating the vertebrae and properly realigning them, they can relieve the stress that misalignment causes to various organs, thus restoring the body to health. Whether the original source of the problem was a misalignment of the spine or distress in an organ, by correcting the misalignment, they can bring relief to the organ. These claims have not been substantiated or proven to the satisfaction of traditional medicine.

## Hypnosis

If you believe in the deep connection between the mind and the body, you may see hypnosis as an avenue for treating your asthma. Hypnosis calls on the resources of your mind to help heal your body—and has proven to be remarkably effective in addressing a wide range of organic conditions (that is, conditions considered to have organic, or physical, causes). For example, a 1988 study at Southampton General Hospital, concerning sixteen patients with chronic asthma, found that after a year of regular hypnosis, the number of times the patients had to be admitted to the hospital fell from forty-four to thirteen, with a concomitant decrease in the length of time they stayed. Six patients were able to stop taking an anti-inflammatory drug altogether, and eight patients were able to get by on reduced dosages. This type of care should be practiced only by a trained and licensed psychologist or psychiatrist!

*What to Expect from Hypnosis* Your actual session should be a relaxing experience. The hypnotist will help you enter a state of deep relaxation, also sometimes called a trance. In this state, you will be more receptive to suggestions that he or she makes, which will help you call up your body's power to heal itself. This process does not depend on either you or the hypnotist believing that your asthma is primarily "psychological" or that your mind is somehow "causing it." Rather, it is based on the idea that the mind can be a powerful ally in helping to heal the body.

In addition to making hypnotic suggestions, a hypnotist may ask questions or help you explore issues that are difficult for you to access in a fully waking state. To the extent that tension, anxiety, and psychological issues are involved in your asthma, even if only as responses to your attacks, hypnosis can be wonderfully calming and relieving.

*Self-Hypnosis* Some hypnotists will work with you to prepare tapes, or to help you prepare tapes, that you can use for self-hypnosis. They may also teach you how to enter a trance whenever you feel an attack coming on, so that you can marshal your body's resources to diffuse the attack. However, there is a *danger that your lungs may be actually worsening, but because your mind is relaxed, you are not aware of that fact.*

*Finding a Hypnotist* If hypnosis interests you, you might turn to hospitals, psychiatric associations, or psychological associations to find a trained hypnotist. Some M.D.s, psychotherapists, psychologists, and psychiatrists have learned to use hypnosis as part of their medical or counseling work. Good hypnotists should be able to explain clearly what they plan to do and why they believe it will work. They should also give you some idea of when to expect results, how many treatments you are likely to need, and what each treatment will cost.

## Visualization

Related to self-hypnosis, visualization is the process of visualizing your body and what you would like to have happen within it. Visualization calls on the powers of the mind to heal the body. Unlike hypnosis, you can explore visualization on your own. People commonly use visualization in two ways: as a regular practice, to promote healing; and when they feel an attack coming on, to ward off the attack.

### Visualization and Tapes

In general, people find tapes very helpful in practicing visualization, particularly the type of tape that can be used as a regular practice. You can make a tape and play it for yourself, or you can find someone whom you love and trust, someone with a soothing voice, to read a prepared script for you. Some health-food stores and alternative bookstores sell visualization and healing tapes.

### Ask Your Doctor about Alternative Treatments

- Do you have any information about alternative treatments that I should be aware of?
- What information would you like to have about my alternative treatments?

### If You are Considering an Alternative "Healer," Ask These Questions:

- How and why does your system work?
- How many treatments/office visits will I need before I can expect results?
- If you are prescribing herbs or other alternative remedies, do I buy them from you? If not, where do I buy them?

- What does a visit cost? What do the herbs or alternative remedies cost?
- Are you covered by insurance?
- What training have you had? What organizations do you belong to? What else should I know about your credentials and your background?

In "Unconventional Therapies in Asthma: An Overview," an article that the journal *Allergy* published in 1996, G. T. Lewith and A. D. Watkins reviewed the evidence for the use of acupuncture, homeopathy, mind-body therapies, and nutritional, herbal, and nutritional medicine in treating asthma. Some of these therapies, the data suggests, seem to benefit patients. Because these techniques are becoming increasingly popular with patients, there is now an urgent need for high-quality research in this area.

# 11

# Working with Your Doctor

Lydia isn't happy with the way things are going with her doctor. She has the feeling that the doctor is too eager to prescribe medication—not concerned enough with her general sense of well-being, not open enough to alternative or holistic approaches, not interested enough in her experience of side effects and other adverse reactions to the medication.

Lydia's first impulse is simply to go along with whatever the doctor says. After all, the doctor has been treating asthma for several years—for far longer than Lydia has been a patient! But Lydia realizes that her dissatisfaction is coming out in small, counterproductive ways. Sometimes she forgets to take her medication. Sometimes she tells the doctor what she thinks is the "right answer" rather than describe her actual condition.

Lydia's second impulse is to leave and find another doctor. But she has been seeing this doctor since she first began to suspect her condition—and she knows that the doctor has an excellent reputation.

Finally, Lydia realizes that she should discuss her concerns with the doctor. That way, the two of them have a chance to improve their relationship. Perhaps she will eventually decide to seek help elsewhere. She hopes, though, that leaving won't be necessary—that she and her doctor can improve communication while improving her treatment.

## Opening the Lines of Communication

Your relationship with your doctor is extremely important, both for your decisions about medication and for your treatment as a whole. That's why this chapter focuses on you and your doctor: knowing what you need from your doctor, getting the most out of each doctor's visit, knowing how to gather the information that your doctor will need, and knowing when to switch doctors. (Understanding the medications your doctor may prescribe is covered in Chapter 12.)

*The Doctor-Patient Relationship: A Two-Way Street* Remember that the doctor-patient relationship has two sides. It's important for you to be clear about what you want from your doctor: advice? comfort? a complete cure? a way of coping with a difficult disease?

Set your sights neither too high ("I want someone who will always be there for me, someone who will cure me completely, someone who can take care of everything for me while handing me the perfect prescription.") nor too low ("He's too busy to explain everything, so I shouldn't complain." "She's not at all interested in nutrition or exercise, but at least she can prescribe an inhaler that works."). You deserve a doctor who will work *with* you to discover the route to health that is best for you, a doctor who both knows the latest research on medication/immunotherapy and is sensitive to issues of nutrition, lifestyle, and general health.

On the other hand, working with a doctor means giving up some of the hope that he or she will turn out to be a godlike creature who dispenses medical advice from Mount Olympus, with no effort or learning necessary on your part.

*Two Points of View* Obviously, you and your doctor approach your illness from very different positions. You have the asthma; the doctor is treating the asthma (unless he or she also has it). You may be hearing information for the first time; the doctor has probably given out this information several times before—if not several hundred times. You may feel scared, on the spot, confused, ashamed, helpless, lonely, or needy; the doctor probably has none of those feelings about treating you (although he or she may certainly feel them at other times, especially when ill). You may have to assimilate a great deal of new information; the doctor is passing on information with which he or she is already familiar.

It's often difficult for doctors to remember what their patients are feeling, to tune in to the experience of the patient. In part, this is because the two types of experience are so different. In part, it's because the doctor may need to keep some emotional distance. If the doctor empathized fully with one dozen or two dozen patients a day, he or she might not be able to treat them all.

In addition, people often hide their distress and confusion, even from sympathetic doctors, in an effort to be "good patients." For example, one patient diligently took notes during a doctor's visit. His physician naturally assumed that the patient was assimilating and recording all the information that the doctor was sharing. On the contrary—the patient's way of handling his anxiety was to write things down. In his view, if he wrote it down, that meant he didn't have to hear it and take it in. He was acting the role of a "good patient" while actually not absorbing a thing. Of course, his doctor had no idea of how frightened he was.

*Treating the Whole Patient*   Many doctors have difficulty dealing with the emotional side of patient care. One thing is certain: If you have asthma, you should be working with a doctor you trust who can prescribe medication. Therefore, it's important that you decide what kind of medical care you want, and that you take steps to get it.

## *Making the Most of an Office Visit*

How can you make every minute of your office visit count? Here are some suggestions:

• *Make a list.* As questions or concerns come to you, jot them down. Before your visit, organize your jottings into a list. This serves three purposes: (1) It will help you focus your thoughts and make sure that you do, in fact, ask all your questions. (2) It will make you a more active, empowered patient, which will help you absorb new information and be more assertive about questioning any new issues that come up during the visit. (3) It will calm you down, which again will make you more empowered and able to care for yourself.

- *Ask about whatever you don't understand.* Many doctors avoid giving patients information—but not always because they're unwilling to share. Some patients don't want information; others think that they want it, but feel frightened or overwhelmed when they get it. If you want to know about something, be assertive and make it clear that this is the kind of doctor-patient relationship you want. If you'd like more information but are nervous about asking for it, role-play a doctor's visit with a friend or spouse, so you can practice asking the kinds of questions you want answered.

- *Take notes.* Despite the example about the note-taking patient who wouldn't listen, taking notes is very important. Besides the obvious benefits of helping you to remember details, it will also help you to feel more empowered and active, and it communicates a strong message to the doctor. Writing something down also gives you a little breathing room during the visit. As you jot down a note, you may realize that you don't fully understand what you're writing. This gives you another chance to ask. Many physicians will give written instructions to you.

- *Write down any new prescriptions.* Make sure you've noted the name of the drug, the strength, when you should take it, how often, and under what restrictions (e.g., not before meals, not with dairy products, and so on). You can use these notes to double-check your pharmacist's printed instructions—and be sure to call the doctor if there is any discrepancy. Furthermore, this note-taking gives you a chance to assimilate the instructions and to ask any questions you may have about them.

- *Repeat the other medications, supplements, and herbs you are taking, as well as any chronic conditions you have.* Even the best doctors sometimes forget things—and even the best patients sometimes forget to pass information on to their doctors. Make sure, each time medication is being discussed, that both your doctor and your pharmacist know about any other medication, even over-the-counter items, that you are already taking. If you suffer from heart disease, blood pressure problems, migraines, or other chronic conditions, remind both your doctor and your pharmacist.

• *Ask whether there are any food restrictions.* This information often is on the patient information sheet that you receive with your medication. If it is not, you should ask your doctor or pharmacist. A food restriction can make a huge difference, both in the intended efficacy of the drug and in your safety.

• *Keep records of how you're doing, bring them with you, and review them with your doctor.* If you're keeping any kind of journal or record, bring it in. Obviously, you won't bring a diary filled with personal observations, but you might review your writing since your last doctor's visit and note any significant good days or bad days, as well as how they related to weather, diet, activity, emotion, and medication. If you're using a peak-flow meter (see the next section), keep a chart of your readings and bring that in. Be assertive; make sure that the doctor knows what's going on with you.

• *Share information about stressful circumstances.* If your symptoms are getting worse and you're going through a divorce, a job upheaval, the loss of a loved one, or any other traumatic event, your doctor should know about it. Stress tends to make all diseases worse, so information about stress in your life should be important to your doctor.

• *If you are having difficulties paying in the way your doctor prefers, bring the matter up and offer to negotiate.* Don't wait until after the visit is over to discuss the bill. The doctor may—understandably—feel taken advantage of and so be less willing to work out an installment plan or other alternative. Tell the doctor what you can about your financial situation, including whether you need him or her to accept Medicare, and make some arrangement that works for both of you.

### *The Peak-Flow Meter: Monitoring Your Own Health*

A peak-flow meter is a device that you can use at home to measure the force with which you are able to exhale at any given point. Often, it's difficult to tell what your breathing capacity is.

Even if you haven't been having symptoms, you may be building up to an attack. A peak-flow meter can help you monitor how your lungs are doing—and a chart of peak-flow meter readings can be invaluable information to share with your doctor. Also, if you and your doctor are working together properly, your peak-flow ratings should improve over time. So measuring your peak flow is also a way of seeing whether your doctor's treatment is doing you any good. It will quite likely be prescribed by your physician, with instructions from the asthma nurse or other personnel.

*Buying a Peak-Flow Meter* A peak-flow meter can be purchased at any drugstore for about $35. It is best to buy a dual-range meter, one that measures both low- and high-range flow rates, because most asthma patients begin in the lower ranges but should expect to progress to the higher ones.

*Using a Peak-Flow Meter*

- Choose the proper range, high or low. (Start with the low range.)
- Stand.
- Inhale as fully as possible.
- Wrap your lips around the mouthpiece of the meter.
- Exhale as hard and as fast as you can.
- Repeat two more times, jotting down each of the three results.
- Compare the three results. Record the best result with the date.

*Taking a Peak-Flow Reading* Ideally, you would take a peak-flow reading each day and at the same time each day, recording the results in your asthma journal or on a separate chart. If that's too demanding or inconvenient, try recording your peak-flow reading twice a day, three times a week. If you are using a bronchodilator, take two sets of readings: one before you inhale the medication, one after (being aware that some medications act quickly and others take thirty minutes to an hour). This will help you see how much difference the medication is making, alerting you to any loss of effectiveness.

Of course, peak-flow readings are no substitute for body awareness. (Other signs of active asthma are a feeling of difficulty moving air, retraction of the spaces between the ribs, and retraction of the spaces above the clavicles.) But the readings can help enhance body awareness, so that your sense of your lungs and their capacity is no longer limited to those moments when you start having symptoms or are in the midst of an attack. Ideally, you will start to be able to feel how much your lungs are improving on the same days that the peak-flow meter registers the improvement.

## When to Consider Changing Doctors

As you think about your relationship with your doctor, you may feel dissatisfied enough to consider changing. Here are some questions that might help you decide whether to take this serious step:

- If you have a question or concern, can you ask your doctor about it?
- If you are not satisfied with some aspect of your treatment, does your doctor take your feeling seriously?
- Do you feel that your doctor is up-to-date on the latest in research on asthma and asthma medications or is willing to refer you to a specialist?
- Does your doctor fully explain what side effects a medication may have, give you clear instructions about what to do in case of side effects, and listen carefully to your reports of your experience with a medication?

*Evaluating the Relationship* The points listed above are the essentials of what you should expect from your doctor. It's possible that, for many reasons, you may decide not to look for the "ideal" doctor who combines emotional sensitivity with up-to-the-minute information, who is able to prescribe medications and to explore alternative methods of healing. In that case, you need to know what aspects of a doctor's abilities are most important to you: a demonstration of care and concern? an ability to return phone calls quickly? a widespread knowledge of medications? a commitment to nutrition and emotional health? You may not find all of your ideal qualities in the same doctor, and you may wish to stay with a doctor who has treated you for a long time and knows you well. You may also have financial or practical reasons for remaining with a particular doctor, depending on your insurance, managed-care, or financial status.

Nevertheless, if you cannot trust your doctor to treat you with respect and to take your concerns seriously, at least as far as prescribing medication and monitoring side effects is concerned, you may need to make other arrangements. A doctor-patient relationship should be characterized by respect and understanding on both sides.

### *Ask Your Doctor . . .*

- Can you take more time to explain to me your reasons for prescribing a particular medication?
- What are the generic and the brand names of the medication?
- Is it possible for me to ask the pharmacist for the generic version, or is there some reason why you are prescribing a particular brand?
- What is your feeling about my exploring nutrition, exercise, breathing exercises, and alternative therapies?

# 12

# Making the Most of the Least Medications

Angela's doctor prescribed an inhaler for her to use in case of an asthma attack. He explained that Angela should take a puff of the albuterol in the inhaler any time she thought an asthma attack might be coming on. He also told her to take a puff before exercise, and then another puff if she felt any ill effects during the exercise itself.

When Angela first got the inhaler, she felt a wonderful sense of freedom and security. At last, she didn't have to worry about asthma attacks! Any time she felt concerned, she could just take a puff of her inhaler and know that the attack would go away.

For the first few weeks, the inhaler worked fine. But then Angela started getting worried. It seems to her that she isn't getting the same relief that she had noticed at first. She also realizes that she is using the inhaler more and more often. She wonders if she should switch to another type of medication—perhaps inhaled steroids, which she has heard are extraordinarily effective and have no side effects. Then Angela reads an article in a magazine about the dangers of steroids, and she worries even more. She wants a medication that will work but that won't endanger her health—and she's starting to think that such a medication just may not exist.

## Work with Your Doctor to Understand Medications

If you've been taking asthma medication for a while, you may be interested in decreasing your reliance on it, even freeing yourself from medication altogether. On the other hand, you may be feeling frustrated with the results you're getting. You may be looking for another, more effective medication. Even if your goal is to reduce your reliance on medication as far as possible, you may need medications available in case of emergency, or you may need to be taking medication for some time before either reducing your dosage or going completely without it.

In either case, you're going to need to work closely with your doctor. Whether you're discontinuing a medication or looking for a new prescription, you should not be acting by yourself. To help you become a more active participant in your own health care, here is some basic information about asthma medication. Work with your doctor to find out more, so that together, the two of you can decide which medication is best for you.

## Categories of Asthma Medications

The two major categories of asthma-related medications are bronchodilators, a quick-relief medication that helps open the airways, and anti-inflammatory drugs, which address the long-term problem of inflammation. Sometimes doctors also prescribe mucokinetic drugs, which help mucus move or clear from the lungs; antihistamines, which also help clear congestion and reduce inflammatory chemicals; and antibiotics, which fight infections when they are needed.

Allergy shots, or immunotherapy, may be considered a medication. It involves the injection, usually on a weekly basis, of tiny doses of the allergen to which you are allergic. There is some danger of an allergic reaction, so these shots should be administered under medical supervision. They can help to turn off the IgE mechanism, with benefits usually within three to six months.

## Bronchodilators

As explained earlier, during an asthma attack, the muscles surrounding the airways constrict. Bronchodilating drugs make constricted muscles dilate, or open, by helping them to relax. In general, bronchodilators are inhaled, although some are taken orally as pills or liquids.

There are three forms of bronchodilators: sympathomimetics (beta-agonists and epinephrine), xanthines (theophylline), and anticholinergics.

### *Beta-Agonists*

Sympathomimetic drugs affect the sympathetic nervous system. The most commonly prescribed drugs in this category are known as the beta-adrenergic agonists, which are also known as beta-adrenergic stimulants, beta-agonists, beta-2 agonists, and beta-2 sympathomimetic agents. These beta-agonists are targeted to stimulate the beta-2 receptors in the lungs, with the goal of getting the receptors to relax bronchial muscles so that the airways open.

Beta-agonists are prescribed in two different ways: to treat symptoms as needed (especially exercise-induced asthma), and to use on a regular schedule (such as once every four, six, eight, or twelve hours) to control chronic asthma. In other words, the person with asthma carries an inhaler and either takes puffs when he or she feels an attack coming on, or takes puffs on a regular schedule determined by a doctor.

Current beta-agonists include albuterol (sold as Proventil and Ventolin); bitolterol (Tornalate), pirbuterol (Maxair), metaproterenol (Alupent, Metaprel), and terbutaline (Brethaire, Brethine, Bricanyl). Salmeterol (Severent) is a beta agent that lasts for twelve hours, but it is categorized as a long-term controller because it should *never* be used more frequently than twice a day, and it should be used only with anti-inflammatory drugs. Sudden respiratory failure has occurred when patients tried to use it in an emergency. Two older beta-agonists, isoetharine (Bronkometer, Bronkosol) and isoproterenol (Isuprel Mistometer) are rarely prescribed, both because they last for shorter periods than the newer beta-agonists and because they have more side effects. An epinephrine (or adrenalin) inhaler is available over the counter as Primatene Mist. It has both alpha- and beta-agonist effects, so it can cause the blood pressure to elevate and the heart to speed up dramatically. It can be useful in a short-term emergency but should not be relied on for regular use.

*Choosing the Right Beta-Agonist*  It often takes doctors and patients a while to figure out which beta-agonist best suits a particular patient. Sometimes this process is simply one of trial and error, as patients discover which drugs work best for them and which have the fewest side effects. The rate of administration is also tailored to the individual according to age. For example, young children tolerate liquid beta-agonists. Patients might also be given metered-dose inhalers, powdered breath-activated inhalers, or long-acting pills.

*Side Effects of Beta-Agonists*  Although beta-agonists prescribed for asthma are targeted at the beta-2 receptors in the muscles of the lungs, they also affect beta-1 receptors in the heart. (Drugs targeted at the heart muscle, with the goal of helping it relax, are known as beta-blockers.) Because of this dual effect, beta-agonists may cause the heart to speed up while blood pressure drops, and along with this, they sometimes cause restlessness, muscle tremors, headaches, and anxiety.

Other possible side effects of beta-agonists include nausea and vomiting. Inhaled forms of the drug seem to cause fewer side effects than oral forms, as inhaled drugs go directly to the lungs, bypassing the bloodstream.

*Masking Inflammation*  The most common problem with beta-agonists is the way in which they mask more serious underlying problems of inflammation. People with asthma may grow used to taking a puff on an inhaler when they feel a problem, not realizing that their airways are becoming more and more inflamed—so that someday the inhaler may not work. Some doctors argue that these fears of severe inflammation are greatly exaggerated, and that they reflect studies done on people with asthma who are more often and more severely ill than most people who have asthma. Other doctors try to steer their patients away from the regular use of beta-agonists and toward more use of antiinflammatory agents, such as cromolyn, nedocromil, or steroids. (For more on steroids, see the section beginning on page 167.)

People with hyperthyroidism, diabetes, or certain types of heart disease should also use bronchodilators only as prescribed.

*When to Call Your Doctor*   Even if you don't have heart disease, if you feel you must take puff after puff of your inhaler to find relief–stop. Call an emergency room or your doctor. By continuing to overuse your inhaler, you are actually taking oxygen away from your heart–the very muscle that needs it most. This could prove fatal.

## *Using Beta-Agonists Effectively*

In general, people who take beta-agonists notice a marvelous relief for the first few weeks. Then, in some cases, people notice far less relief over time. Sometimes the drop in effectiveness is because the airways have simply become less responsive to the drug. In other cases, people are simply not shaking their canisters properly, so that they get a good-size dose when the container is full and a smaller one when it starts to empty. Also, it is not easy to tell when the medication is used up, because the canister may continue to spray.

A common cause of side effects is to let the spray settle on the tongue, where it can be swallowed and make its way into the bloodstream, rather than inhaling correctly or using a spacer device to direct more into the lungs. Some patients find that if they rinse their mouths out after spraying, they experience far fewer side effects.

*Cutting Back on Beta-Agonists*   If you are interested in reducing your use of inhalers and beta-agonists, *work with your doctor*. It is often possible, when you have improved your avoidance measures, nutrition, exercise, and breathing habits, to reduce your use of bronchodilators dramatically. Many patients use them only when they feel an acute attack coming on. Moreover, if you are using a peak-flow meter, you may realize that there are times when you think you need a spray, but when your lungs are actually functioning quite well.

*Use Your Inhaler Correctly* Here are some suggestions for using metered-dose inhalers most effectively. If you've been using one for quite a while, you may feel that this procedure has become second nature—but pause and consider. A recent study of asthma patients found that few used these sprays correctly. New types of inhalers are available and the proper use will vary. Be sure that you have instructions.

**Suggestions for Using Metered-Dose Inhalers**

*Without a Spacer Device*

1. Shake the canister well.
2. Open your mouth.
3. Breathe out.
4. Put the canister about an inch from your mouth, holding it level.
5. Spray toward the back of your throat. Remember, your goal is your lungs, not your tongue.
6. As you spray, take a deep breath in.
7. Hold your breath for ten seconds, to allow the spray to work its way throughout your lungs. Then exhale.
8. If you have been prescribed two puffs, remember that each puff is a separate dose of medicine. Wait about five minutes between each one.
9. Clean your container after use, so that dust and particles don't contaminate your spray. This is equally important if you are using the new chlorofluorocarbon (CFC)-free inhaler, Proventil HFA. Because the spray contains finer particles the opening from the canister is smaller, and it must be washed at least weekly. Of course, keep your container covered when you're not using it.
10. If you're in the midst of an acute attack, wait about fifteen minutes before taking a second dose from the

inhaler. This can be a long, frustrating wait, but it will give your lungs a chance to respond to the first dose, making the second dose even more effective.

*With a Spacer Device*

A spacer—a tube of various shapes—attaches to the mouthpiece of the canister. (You can get one at your drugstore with a prescription.) The spacer increases the space between the canister and your mouth and acts as a reservoir.

1. Place the mouthpiece into your mouth.
2. Activate the inhaler and breathe in *slowly* and *deeply* several times before removing it from your mouth. Some devices have a whistle that sounds if you are breathing too fast.

*Breath-Activated Inhalers*

More of these inhalers, such as Maxair, will be available as metered-dose inhalers containing CFC (chlorofluorocarbon) are phased out. A child under the age of six rarely can use this type successfully.

1. Shake the inhaler.
2. Put your mouth on the inhalator and take a *fast* deep breath.
3. Hold the breath for twenty seconds.

## *Epinephrine*

Another type of sympathomimetic drug is epinephrine, or adrenaline (Adrenalin, Epipen), which is generally used only in emergencies. Primatene Mist, which is available over the counter, contains epinephrine, which may give transient relief, but which is very short-acting and should not be relied upon. As mentioned in Chapter 4, people who suffer from allergies may carry an EpiPen or other source of injectable epinephrine for use in case of anaphylactic shock.

### Theophylline

This drug is used less frequently since newer medications are available. Common xanthines, also known as methylxanthines, include theophylline (Aerolate, Quibron, Respbid, Slo-Bid, Theo-Dur) and aminophylline (available in intravenous or pill form), a kind of theophylline given intravenously only. In most popular literature, this category of drug is simply referred to as theophylline.

These drugs relax bronchial muscles, reduce respiratory muscle fatigue, and may combat inflammation. However, they also stimulate the central nervous system and the heart (much as caffeine does). Theophylline used in combination with inhaled beta-agonists has an even greater bronchodilating effect than either drug used alone.

Theophylline is usually taken as a pill or syrup. It's a difficult drug to manage, because if the amount of it in your bloodstream is too low, it has no effect, whereas if the amount is too high, it may produce severe adverse reactions (which should be reported to a doctor *immediately*): nausea, vomiting, stomachache, loss of appetite, irregular heartbeat, severe headache, confusion, disorientation, and seizure. Even when used properly, theophylline may cause irritability, restlessness, and sleeping difficulties.

*Monitoring Theophylline* If you're taking theophylline, your doctor needs to monitor the amount of theophylline in your blood at least every six months—more often until levels are stabilized, or if you start feeling side effects, if the theophylline doesn't seem to be working, or if you have any condition that may alter the way you metabolize (break down) the theophylline. These conditions include fevers, viral infection, liver disease, heart disease, flu vaccines, and some drugs, including erythromycin (an antibiotic), ulcer drugs such as cimetidine, heart medications, and birth-control pills. These factors cause your body to metabolize theophylline more slowly, so you need less of it—and are therefore in more danger of an overdose.

Patients who have serious liver problems should certainly avoid theophylline, which passes through the liver. If the liver is not properly metabolizing the drug, it stays at high levels in the bloodstream and can soon become toxic.

*Interactions of Theophylline with Other Medications* Theophylline interacts with many other medications—and with the caffeine in your morning tea or coffee. Because both theophylline and caffeine speed up your system, you may be suffering from toxic effects even if the actual levels of theophylline in your blood are acceptable.

Here's a list of common substances that interfere with theophylline, causing it to be metabolized either slower or faster than normal:

### Substances That Interfere with Theophylline

*Increased Metabolism*

- *Smoke.* If you smoke, you're metabolizing this drug at twice the rate of a nonsmoker, so you need a higher-than-average dose.
- *Protein.* If you're on a high-protein, low-carbohydrate diet, you metabolize theophylline at a 25 percent faster rate than normal.
- *Nicotine.* This drug increases theophylline metabolism and may necessitate very high doses to be effective.
- *Phenytoin.* An anticonvulsant, this drug works less well when theophylline is present, and it increases the metabolism, thus lowering the level of theophylline.

*Decreased Metabolism*

- *Carbohydrates.* If you are on a low-protein, high-carbohydrate diet, you will metabolize theophylline 25 percent more slowly than the average person.
- *Infection.* During any type of viral infection or fever, your body will metabolize theophylline more slowly.
- *Caffeine.* Coffee, tea, chocolate, and caffeinated drinks add to the side effects of theophylline.
- *Inderal.* This commonly prescribed heart medication slows the metabolism of theophylline, so you'll need a lower dose of theophylline if you are taking both drugs.

- *Some antibiotics.* Such drugs as erthyromycin and the class of antibiotics known as quinolones–both of which are prescribed for people who have both asthma and respiratory infections–can decrease the metabolism and thereby increase the blood levels of theophylline.
- *Cimetidine.* Sold as Tagamet, this ulcer medication decreases metabolism of theophylline and increases serum levels.
- *Vaccines.* Flu vaccines interfere with metabolism of theophylline.

In addition, theophylline increases the elimination of lithium (often prescribed for manic-depression) from the body.

*Evaluating Theophylline* For many patients, theophylline is a useful drug. For anyone who takes it, however, there is an ever-present risk of side effects, adverse reactions, and problems with metabolism. If you and your doctor decide to go with this medication, be sure that you understand how to monitor your own health and how to keep your doctor informed.

## *Anticholinergics*

The third type of bronchodilator is the anticholinergic drugs, also known as the parasympatholytics, which work on the parasympathetic nervous system. Atropine, the first such drug developed in this category, is rarely prescribed any more because of its side effects. However, ipratropium bromide (Atrovent) is often prescribed, in inhaled form. It acts more slowly than beta-agonists–it takes an hour to reach peak effectiveness, as opposed to albuterol's average of five minutes–but once it begins to work it lasts longer. It is frequently added to beta-agonists as a second-line bronchodilator. It is said to work best with asthma precipitated by viral infections, gastroesophageal reflux, or emotional triggers. It is also effective for chronic bronchitis.

Possible side effects of ipratropium bromide include dry mouth, palpitations, and, occasionally, difficulties with urination. It may also make glaucoma worse. A metered-dose inhaler that combines albuterol and ipratropium (combinent) is now available.

## Anti-Inflammatory Drugs

The latest weapons in the asthma arsenal are various types of anti-inflammatory drugs. These have proved enormously popular with many doctors and patients, particularly because they have a prophylactic (preventive) role, rather than merely responding to symptoms. Most doctors believe that if you need to use a bronchodilator more than a few times a week (mild persistent asthma, according to the guidelines on page 36), you should also be taking anti-inflammatory drugs, to work on the long-term effects of chronic asthma. There is good evidence that people who take anti-inflammatory drugs are far less likely to respond to asthma triggers.

Four major types of anti-inflammatory drugs are available: cromolyn sodium, nedocromil, corticosteroids, and leukotriene modifiers.

### *Steroids*

Corticosteroids, also known as steroids, are receiving good reviews from many doctors and patients, who credit this type of medication with enabling them to live virtually normal lives, with far less responsiveness to asthma triggers. Nevertheless, some patients report side effects from inhaled steroids—and many doctors are concerned about the long-term, cumulative effects of this type of medication. Many of us remember all too well the successive waves of "fashionable" medications that are at first greeted with enthusiasm and then prove to cause unforeseen problems, only to be superseded by a new generation of "latest discoveries." This is not to say that you should avoid inhaled steroids, only that they, like other medications, have profound effects on your body.

There are two ways that steroids are prescribed for asthma patients: to be taken orally, and to be inhaled. The inhaled form allows for far lower doses since the medication is delivered directly to the airways if it is administered correctly.

*How Steroids Work* Both oral and inhaled steroids are potent medications. So let's begin by looking at what steroids are and how they work. Steroids are naturally produced by the body's adrenal glands. They serve many functions in the body, including helping us to metabolize sugars and fats and regulating inflammation. When scientists first discovered how to synthesize steroids in the laboratory, these potent synthetic substances were hailed as a new miracle drug.

*Side Effects of Steroids* The long-term use of oral or injected steroids seems to disrupt virtually every organ in the body, in many cases, causing long-term irreversible harm. Steroids force nutrients out of cells at a much faster rate than normal, which means that a person taking steroids is losing minerals that he or she needs for normal functioning, particularly potassium, calcium, and magnesium. The result: electrolyte imbalances, nutritional deficiencies, and the related problems that they cause, including a depressed immune system, poor healing of wounds, weight gain, changes in the metabolism of fat, high blood pressure, osteoporosis (thinning of the bones), thinning of the skin, damage to the heart and lungs, pain in the joints, bleeding in the stomach, severe acne, extra hair growth, cataracts, mood disorders, and in some cases, psychosis. People who use steroids daily for long periods often notice a swelling of the face and ankles.

*Long-Term Steroid Use* The long-term use of steroids can impair the functioning of the adrenal glands. As the pituitary glands that stimulate the adrenals recognize the artificially high level of this substance in the bloodstream, they shut off their own hormone production. Over time, the adrenals may actually shrink.

Doctors debate whether short-term and low-dose steroid therapies, including the milder therapy of inhaled steroids, pose any risk of these side effects. As with all medications, there are probably wide variations, and there is probably a great deal yet unknown about long-term effects. Studies have shown that at least some people are affected adversely even by inhaled steroids, especially if given in high doses, suffering from the major side effects associated with all steroids: adrenal suppression, osteoporosis, cataracts, and the like.

People taking inhaled steroids may also get thrush, a fungal infection of the mouth. This can often be avoided by rinsing the mouth after each inhalation, and by using a spacer device. Sometimes people cough or have a creaky voice after the inhalation, but these symptoms tend to be temporary.

### When to Use Steroids

Even with all the precautions, there are definitely times when steroids are the best available treatment. (For more on steroids and children, see Chapter 13.) Here is the latest available information on inhaled and oral steroids.

*Inhaled Steroids* Inhaled steroids currently on the market include beclomethasone (Beconase, Beclovent, Vanenase, Vanceril), flunisolide (AeroBid, Nasalide), triamcinolone (Azmacort, Nasacort), budesonide (Pulmocort), and fluticasone (Flovent).

If you're taking inhaled steroids, don't expect results right away. It takes from one to four weeks for this type of medication to kick in. After that, lungs become less "twitchy" and hyperresponsive. Bearing the earlier warnings in mind, also note that most patients *seem* to experience very few side effects from inhaled steroids, particularly if used correctly.

*Oral Steroids* Oral steroids are used when inhaled steroids aren't powerful enough, as in the case of a severe asthma attack. In this case, a doctor might prescribe short-term steroid therapy with such oral or injectable steroids as dexamethasone (Decadron), methylprednisolone (Medrol), prednisone (Deltasone), and triamcinolone (Aristocort). The goal of such short-term therapy—say, one dose per day for three to ten days—is to stop the severe inflammation that can result when the asthma attack is underway.

Sometimes, too, doctors prescribe oral steroids on a long-term basis, for people with severe chronic asthma. However, the long-term use of oral corticosteroids can suppress the body's normal production of hormones. In some cases, doctors prescribe oral steroids for every other day, rather than daily, to reduce the likelihood of adrenal suppression.

The advantage of oral steroids is that they work quickly and thoroughly, with relief beginning in three hours and peaking in six to twelve hours. The disadvantage—and it's a major one—is the side effects. Long-term ill effects include cataracts (a clouding of the lens of the eye that blocks vision), osteoporosis (loss of bone mass) with spontaneous vertebral fractures, high blood pressure, diabetes, and an impaired immune system.

If this information about corticosteroids is of concern to you, talk it over with your doctor. *Never discontinue oral steroids without a doctor's supervision.* Your body could go into shock from suddenly stopping their use. If you have been taking oral steroids for more than a short period of time you should wear a medic-alert bracelet or dog tag indicating such use.

*Timing Your Use of Steroids* Steroids are naturally produced by the body just after waking; in most people, steroids are at their lowest levels between 2 A.M. and 4 A.M. So if you take steroids first thing in the morning, you are supporting your body's natural functioning, and your brain will be less likely to interpret high levels of steroids in the bloodstream as a reason to shut off your adrenal glands' own functioning. On the other hand, if you suffer from nighttime asthma, you may need to take your steroids before bedtime. Some recent studies suggest that three o'clock in the afternoon is the best time to take steroids. In any case, however, try—with your doctor's supervision—to take steroids only once during twenty-four hours, rather than in divided doses. Short-acting steroids such as prednisone are less likely to cause adrenal suppression.

*Compensating for Steroids* Here's a list of some of the nutrients and minerals that you may need to replace while you are using steroids, either oral or inhaled. As always, work with your doctor when taking vitamin, mineral, and other supplements:

**Nutrients Lost from Steroid Use**

- *Potassium.* The loss of potassium, known as hypokalemia, can lead to congestive heart failure and heart irregularities. Symptoms of this condition include muscle weakness (the first sign), and eventual muscle paralysis (including the muscles around the lungs). Work with your physician to monitor potassium, because either too much or too little produces toxic effects.

- *Protein.* It's the loss of protein that produces the side effects of loss of muscle mass. This only occurs with prolonged high-dose therapy. A high-protein diet, rich in fish, milk, soy, and, in some cases, protein supplements, can compensate for this effect.
- *Calcium and magnesium.* These two minerals work as a team, each displacing the other within your cells. The balance of these two minerals is crucial for the healthy functioning of your system. You may be able to address this issue by taking calcium citrate, magnesium citrate, and/or magnesium aspartate—under a doctor's care, of course. (Be careful: Too much magnesium can cause diarrhea.)

### *Cromolyn Sodium and Nedocromil*

Cromolyn sodium (also called sodium cromoglycate) is an anti-inflammatory drug that is different from steroids. Sold under the name Intal, this drug seems to stabilize mast cells and other cells, preventing them from releasing the inflammatory chemicals that cause asthma attacks.

Cromolyn seems to prevent airways from narrowing in response to exercise, cold air, sulfur dioxide, and pollen, though it must be taken at least fifteen minutes before exposure to these triggers. Once an attack has begun, cromolyn is not very effective; a bronchodilator works better. The main benefit of cromolyn is that it seems to prevent exercise-induced asthma, as well as allergen-induced asthma. However, some asthma patients simply don't respond to it. People who do respond well to cromolyn often take it from two to four times a day as part of a maintenance program. If you're interested in trying this medication, be prepared to give it up to a month to see whether it works for you.

Side effects of cromolyn include rare wheezing or coughing. Because side effects are so few and so mild, doctors often choose this medication for patients with mild asthma. It may be used as a metered-dose inhaler or as a solution in a jet nebulizer, with or without added bronchodilator.

A similar drug, nedocromil sodium (Tilade), available as a metered-dose inhaler, is often prescribed in similar situations and is more potent than cromolyn. Again, there are no side effects other than a bad taste that some people experience. Some feel that nedocromil is especially effective for the cough associated with asthma.

### *Leukotriene Modifiers*

Leukotrienes are potent mediators of prolonged asthma that are formed and released from cell membranes during the allergic or asthmatic reaction. Three new medications are now available to combat leukotrienes, and these drugs may be used in place of other anti-inflammatory agents. Initial studies have shown efficacy in patients with mild persistent asthma, and physicians are now trying them in patients with more severe asthma to see if they can help reduce the need for high-dose or systemic corticosteroids. Some patients who have required oral steroids for many years have responded well but have developed a severe cosinophilic pneumonia, so doctors are being urged to exericse caution in taking patients off steroids if they have used them for a long time.

The new drugs include Zileuton (Zyflo), a tablet that must be taken four times a day and is approved for use by people older than twelve (users must have blood tests for liver enzyme function performed regularly); Zafirlukast (Accolate), which is approved for people older than twelve and is taken twice a day on an empty stomach; and Monteleukast (Singular), which is available as a chewable tablet, taken once daily, and approved for children as young as six.

## Mucokinetic Drugs

This type of drug helps to clear mucus from the lungs. The medication known as guaifenesin, an expectorant (which helps people cough, or expectorate, mucus from the lungs) is found in many cough and cold syrups. Doctors sometimes prescribe it for asthma, to help the patient cough up more mucus. There are few side effects other than nausea and vomiting. A more potent drug is iodinated glycerol (Organidin). Side effects of these drugs include nausea, vomiting, and goiter if used long-term.

Some lower-intensity mucokinetic treatments are also available, such as saltwater solutions that are sprayed into the nostrils. Hot, steamy liquids, such as chicken soup and tea, and garlic, may also be helpful.

## Antihistamines

This type of drug relieves nasal congestion and sneezing, as well as hives that may result from an allergic reaction. One of the effects of histamine is bronchospasm. Certainly, histamine is present in high concentrations in the bloodstream during an attack—as well as during times when a person with asthma is responsive to allergens. The newer nonsedating antihistamines do not have anticholergenic effects, which cause thickening of mucus, so they are frequently helpful in patients with asthma due to allergy.

## Allergy Shots

Allergy shots (allergen immunotherapy) involve the administration of very small doses of extracts of allergens to which a patient has reacted positively in a skin test. The allergens given in shots are those that appear to cause significant symptoms and cannot be avoided—for example, pollen, molds, and dust mites. The shots are usually given once or twice a week in the build-up phase, and then they are spaced out to once every two or three weeks. This is the only method known to decrease hyperactivity other than prolonged avoidance of the allergens. There is some risk of reaction to the shots, ranging from mild local reactions to severe reactions including wheezing, hives, or even shock. Therefore it is strongly recommended that the shots be administered only when medical caregivers are nearby, and that patients wait at least twenty to thirty minutes after the injection. Patients usually notice improvement within three to six months of the beginning of the therapy. Shots should never be given to a patient who is already having an asthmatic attack.

Experiments with immunotherapy administered orally and even nasally are underway, but these methods have not yet been approved by the FDA.

## Finding the Medication That Works for You

For people with asthma, medication can be a double-edged sword. On the one hand, it brings security, safety, and relief from symptoms. On the other hand, it might cause side effects—and if medication does not work, patients can feel doubly frightened.

This double-edge sword requires a double-edged approach. First, of course, *work with your doctor.* Keep him or her informed of how your medication is affecting you and what concerns you have. Second, remain aware—of your body, your feelings, your attitude. In the final analysis, you are the expert on how your medication is affecting you.

*Ask Your Doctor ...*

- How long should I expect to use this medication before my symptoms are relieved?
- What should I do if I don't experience any relief?
- What side effects should I expect?
- Which side effects warrant a call to your office?
- Which side effects mean that I should immediately stop taking the medication?
- Which side effects mean that I should go right to the emergency room?
- How often should I take this medication?
- Is there a particular time of day I should be taking it?

- How much should I take?
- What happens if I forget a dose?
- Do I take this medication with meals or on an empty stomach?
- Will this medication interact with the other prescription drugs I am taking?
- Will it interact with the other over-the-counter drugs I am taking?
- Will it interact badly with any particular foods?
- Will it interact badly with any vitamin supplements or mineral supplements?
- What about long-term use of this medication? What are the possible long-term effects?
- How long do you anticipate that I will need to take this medication?
- Are there steps we could take to reduce my dosage or to free me from it entirely?
- Can I look forward to getting off medication entirely? To reducing it considerably? What is your prognosis?
- What should I do about my allergy shots if I am sick?

# 13

# Children and Asthma: What Every Parent Needs to Know

Paul's family realizes that they all have to make some changes. Paul is becoming more and more fearful, frustrated, and isolated. Because his asthma has become such a big part of his life, he, his family, and his friends are starting to feel that his asthma *is* his life; that his entire personality is dominated by the condition of having asthma.

Paul's parents take three major steps:

1. They make changes in Paul's diet and home environment that should help him avoid the substances that were contributing to his hypersensitive airways.
2. They work with his doctor to find out about the kinds of exercise that Paul can do, and then they work with Paul to help him become more physically active and to find preventive medications with few side effects.
3. They have a few sessions with a family counselor, who helps Paul, his siblings, and his parents learn ways of talking through their feelings, about Paul's asthma and about other issues, so that everyone in the family feels better about themselves and each other.

These steps don't solve everything. Both Paul and the other members of his family still feel frustrated with Paul's asthma at times. There are still things Paul can't do, still ways that his asthma interferes with his life. But things have gotten so much better that Paul and everyone else in his family are now much more hopeful. They can imagine that both Paul's life and family life in general will continue to improve.

## Asthma: A Family Issue

Childhood asthma affects some 4 million children in the United States. Of all the emergency room and hospital admissions, of all the missed school days caused by chronic childhood illnesses, asthma causes the most.

### Childhood Asthma: A Disease on the Rise

The incidence of childhood asthma continues to increase. During the 1970s, the prevalence of asthma in the United States increased by 58 percent among children aged six to eleven. From 1981 to 1988, asthma among U.S. children under age eighteen increased by another 40 percent. Asthma remains 26 percent higher in African American children than in white children, and 12 percent higher in all children who live in households with incomes below the poverty level.

*Widespread Effects* The effects of childhood asthma are not limited to the children who suffer from it. The disease also affects those children's families: the mothers and fathers who sit up nights with children laboring to breathe, who take them to the emergency room, who arrange for time off from their jobs to care for a child who is sick, who call the schools and try to make yet another arrangement for missed school time. And childhood asthma affects the brothers and sisters of the child with asthma, who watch their sibling suffer, who see their own trips and birthday parties and play dates with friends disrupted, who see their worried parents direct what seems like extra attention to the sick child, who have their own fears and questions about their own health as well as their responsibilities to their "sick" brother or sister.

### *Parental Responsibility*

Parents of children with asthma have three sets of responsibilities. First, they need to find out as much as they can about the disease and its treatment. They need to know not just the information covered in the earlier chapters of this book—what causes asthma, how to minimize or avoid asthma triggers, how to work with a doctor—but also the specifics of how that information affects children, particularly what medications are or are not recommended for childhood use and how to "asthma-proof" their child's room and the entire home as far as possible.

Second, parents need to work with their child to help him or her cope with the disease. Together, they need to explore what patterns of diet and exercise, what negotiations with friends and school, will work for their child. Parents need to decide when they themselves should intervene—as in protesting the regulations that don't allow children to carry an inhaler—and when to let the children speak for themselves.

Finally, parents need to see asthma as a *family* problem, one that affects every single member of the family. They need to find ways that every family member can express his or her feelings about the asthma that is affecting everybody.

The good news is that by seeing asthma as a family problem, the resources of the entire family can be marshaled to solve it. Helping the child with asthma take responsibility for his or her own health can take some of the burden off the parents. Finding a way that every family member can express his or her feelings means that everyone gets along better and can pitch in more.

### *The Warning Signs of Childhood Asthma*

Let's start at the beginning. How do you know if your child has asthma?

## Symptoms of Childhood Asthma

- Wheezing
- Coughing
- Shortness of breath
- Chest tightness
- Rapid breathing
- Intolerance of exercise
- Itchy, watery eyes
- Stuffy, runny nose
- Sore throat
- Dark circles under the eyes
- Flared nostrils
- Labored breathing
- Hunched posture

## Symptoms in Infants with Asthma

- Refusal to suck
- Continuous coughing
- Wheezing
- "Fussy" behavior
- Blue color around mouth or nails

Obviously, any of the symptoms listed above may be caused by conditions other than asthma.

## Conditions That Mimic Asthma in Children

- Croup—an infectious disease common in children aged three months to three years, associated with noisy breathing on inspiration. May be recurrent in allergic children.
- Epiglottitis—an inflammation of the epiglottis, the cap that keeps food from entering the windpipe. This is usually associated with high fever, refusal to eat, drooling.

- Cystic fibrosis—a hereditary disease of the lungs and pancreas. May present with cough and wheezing
- Pneumonia—an inflammation of the lungs
- Bronchitis—an acute disease of the breathing tubes marked by frequent coughing
- Bronchiolitis—an inflammation of the lining of the small airways, or bronchioles, which both resembles asthma and may herald its coming. Respiratory Syvettial Virus (RSV) infections are commonly called bronchiolitis.

*Working with Your Pediatrician* If your child has any of these conditions, discuss the appropriate tests and diagnoses with your doctor. Work with your doctor to determine as well if any of these conditions might help bring on asthma, especially if there is a history of asthma in your family.

### *Childhood vs. Adult Asthma: Answers to Your Questions*

There are many myths and half-truths about childhood asthma that can interfere with a full understanding of your child and his or her condition. At the same time, medical knowledge of asthma is changing so quickly that the answers to these questions are also changing. Here is the latest medical thinking on the most common questions about childhood asthma:

*When Are Children Likely to First Develop Asthma?* Most childhood asthma develops between the ages of two and five, although some infants also show signs of asthma. However, childhood asthma generally develops in response to the presence of IgE antibodies that react to allergens (see Chapter 2 for more information). It usually takes a few years before children build up these antibodies. This is good to know, because if there is a history of asthma or allergy in your family, you can use the early years of your child's infancy to develop a home environment that contains as few allergy triggers as possible (see suggestions on page 183).

*Do Most Children "Outgrow" Asthma?* In the past, childhood asthma was seen as a disease that was automatically outgrown; and indeed, this seemed to be the case. In the past two decades, however, fewer and fewer children have spontaneously outgrown their asthma. In some cases, asthma may go away by itself. In other cases, it may only seem to disappear, during, say, the teen years, only to recur more forcefully in a person's twenties or thirties. In still other cases, the asthma does not disappear—in fact, it may grow worse.

Children who do seem to outgrow asthma tend to do so at one of two stages: after age six or in their teenage years, both times when smaller airways increase in size. About 50 percent of children whose asthma began between ages two and eight escape asthma during their teens and twenties—but about half of those develop asthma again in their late twenties or early thirties. Because doctors don't know which children are likely to outgrow their asthma and which will not, you and your doctor need to make sure your child's asthma is effectively treated. Avoiding allergens and irritants helps decrease bronchial hyperreactivity at any age. Allergy prick tests, when properly done, can be helpful in identifying allergens at any age.

## Courses of Action

Knowing about the speed and intensity of childhood asthma attacks points to two important courses of action: eliminating as many allergens and asthma triggers as possible from your child's environment, and working with your child to find safe and pleasant ways for him or her to exercise. You should also have an action plan so that you and the child know what to do if an attack begins and also if it worsens.

### *Creating a Safe Environment for Your Child*

Every parent wants to create a safe environment for his or her child. Parents of children with asthma, however, have an even greater stake in removing allergens and irritants from their child's home. Not only does removing these lessen the possibility of an attack caused by a substance in the home, but lowering the number of allergens and irritants that your child encounters helps to generally lower his or her threshold of allergic reaction. For example, if your child encounters ten allergens in a single day, he or she may generally react less intensely to any one of them than if he or she encounters fifty or a hundred allergens. (To see how every exposure to an allergen/asthma trigger raises the stakes for a person with asthma, take another look at Chapters 3, 4, and 5.)

*Cigarette Smoke—the Single Greatest Asthma Trigger* Every child is different, and an environmental trigger that may adversely affect one child with asthma—say, household dust—may have virtually no impact on another child. However, virtually all children react with intensely negative effects to cigarette smoke.

Study after study has verified that children with asthma who live in homes where one or more people smoke are far more likely to suffer asthma attacks than children who live in nonsmoking homes. According to James E. Haddow, M.D., of the Foundation of Blood Research, as quoted in the *Medical Tribune* of July 8, 1993, "If parents of asthmatic children would stop smoking, it could cut the number of times their children have to seek medical help for asthma attacks by up to 80 percent."

If you or your spouse smoke, it can be tempting to think that you can smoke at home as long as you do so when your child isn't in the room. Unfortunately, cigarette smoke lingers long after the smoker has finished, presenting your child with an ever-present asthma trigger. To fully protect your child, you, your spouse, and all other adults who live in your home have to commit to giving up smoking entirely—or at least to smoking far away from home.

**Protect Your Child from Smoke**

- Don't let *anyone* smoke in your home, whether relatives, formal guests, or such visitors as repair people and delivery people.
- Don't allow your children to carpool or ride with neighbors or relatives who routinely smoke while driving. (Remember that cigarette smoke is present in the car even when the driver isn't smoking.)
- Find out whether your children's friends live with adults who smoke. If they do, find alternative places for your

child to play with that friend, explaining the situation to the children and parents involved.

*Removing Other Household Environmental Triggers* For more ideas on how to asthma-proof your house, take another look at Chapter 6. In addition, here are some of the most important ways that you can protect your child from asthma triggers in his or her bedroom. The bedroom is emphasized because this is usually where the child spends the most consecutive hours. (If the child has had allergy prick tests, you may know more specifically the exact allergens to be avoided.)

- Reduce dust by covering mattresses and pillows with vinyl or impermeable casings. Inexpensive ones can be obtained from most department stores, but they dry out and crack within a few months. Slightly more expensive ones made of vinyl-polyester are very comfortable and can be obtained from several sources. (By the way, with a doctor's prescription, these can be a tax-deductible medical expense.)
- If allergic to home dust mites, wash all sheets once a week in temperatures of at least 130°F to kill dust mites. If you are concerned about having the water temperature so high, you can use a dryer on an extra-high setting, which may accomplish the task.
- Find vinyl or plastic toys rather than traditional stuffed animals for your child. Some are stuffed with polyester and are washable. If necessary, have your child's stuffed animals "sleep in another room." Periodically placing a stuffed animal in a plastic bag and placing it in the freezer overnight can kill dust mites.
- Keep your child's room as free as possible from books, toys, and other items that might collect dust.
- If possible, remove carpets from your child's room. If that's not possible, vacuum them every week and shampoo them every month.
- Whether you are vacuuming carpets or floors, you can use a special high-quality vacuum made for people with aller-

gies, which contains a HEPA filter such as Nilfisk, Vita-Vac, and Euroclean. Although most vacuum cleaners stir up dust, these special models collect dust. Alternatively, supplement your regular vacuum cleaner with a specially designed filter or double bags made to trap dust that would be emitted into the room.

- Replace heavy drapes or venetian blinds with curtains, shades, or shutters that you can wash frequently.
- Every week, wipe woodwork, closets, drawers, and other dust-collecting surfaces with a damp cloth.
- Keep humidity at a level between 35 percent and 40 percent. If you use a humidifier or dehumidifier to achieve this air quality, make sure that you clean the machine regularly to prevent mold growth.
- Replace standard filters in your forced-air heating system with electrostatic air precipitators, which will filter and clean the air in your child's bedroom, keeping it free from dust, mold spores, and pollen. (You can get these special filters from air-conditioner distributors.)
- Clean all air ducts in your home, and keep them clean. Have them cleaned professionally if problems continue.
- If necessary, buy a room-size HEPA filter for your child's bedroom. (For more on HEPA filters, see Chapter 6.)
- Minimize fuzzy or stuffed toys.
- Do not allow smokers into the house.
- Keep the bedroom uncarpeted.
- Do not use talcum powder or perfumed lotions.
- Do not allow pets indoors.
- Avoid wool blankets and feather pillows or comforters.

*Addressing Asthma through Diet*

Many of the suggestions about diet in Chapter 8 will work for your child. Both children and adults benefit from an allergen-free diet if they are allergic to specific foods or if prick tests have suggested a food allergy. If you are not sure whether the foods are truly allergenic, you can experiment with a one-week trial, eliminating all foods that you suspect of causing problems. (Eliminating one food at a time may not help because your child may continue to be exposed to numerous other allergens.) Go on to reintroduce one "suspect" food at a time, every two days, watching closely for an increase in symptoms. Do not do this at home if the child has previously had anaphylaxis, hives, or severe asthma with a food.

Babies should be breast-fed if possible, and they should be introduced to new foods slowly.

Milk, peanuts, eggs, tomatoes, and soy (found in many products as a filler) are common allergens for children as well as for adults, and they form the basis for many children's diets. Remember, your child is more likely to become allergic to the foods that he or she is most often exposed to, so you might also work with your child to vary his or her diet as much as possible.

Avoiding certain foods even temporarily can be more difficult with children than with adults. (Giving up or cutting back on a favorite food can be hard enough for adults!) It may help to enlist the child's help as far as possible. For example, suppose that you need to establish an allergen-freed diet for your daughter. You could begin by telling her that you are going to play "food detective," to figure out which foods make her feel better and which might give her allergies. If she's old enough, have her help you make a chart to keep track of what she's eaten and when she ate it. If possible, involve her in keeping an asthma journal to record her reactions to food (as well as to other possible asthma triggers). The more your daughter feels responsible for her own health, the more cooperative she's likely to be in doing the things that will make her feel better and keep her healthy.

Remember that even if an asthma attack occurs after your child has eaten a certain food, it might have occurred by chance or been caused by factors other than the food. Help your child to keep a positive, cheerful attitude about food and eating, rather than to fear eating because it is linked to allergies.

You must work with a doctor to discover the diet that is best for your child. Allergy prick tests done by a well-trained allergist or immunologist can be very useful in guiding a trial diet or in suggesting foods that should be eliminated for a trial period or for a longer period of time. Those tests rarely cause any symptoms and can be placed on the arm or back very quickly, while the child is distracted with games or videos. It is sad to see children suffer for several years because parents or primary care physicians fear testing or do not understand how useful it can be. Prick tests have also been helpful in differentiating between diary and soy allergies in infants.

## *Building Good Exercise Habits*

As discussed earlier, exercise can be especially painful for children with asthma. Without necessarily knowing why, a child with asthma may avoid the activity that eventually results in a tight chest, a painful sensation in the lungs, or a shortness of breath, let alone a full-blown asthma attack.

You can solve this problem, although again, it may take patience and creativity. As always, start with your doctor. Find out what he or she thinks your child can do. (If your doctor advises against all forms of exercise, you might seriously consider whether you want to find another doctor.)

*Creating an Exercise Plan with Your Child*   After consulting with your doctor, work with your child to create an exercise program that feels fun and safe. First review what your child can do to cope with any asthma attack that is triggered by exercise. Your child can learn many if not all of the breathing exercises in Chapter 9, as well as develop his or her own visualization and self-hypnosis techniques for calming down and restoring normal breathing during an attack (see Chapter 10). Preventive medications, whether liquid, tablets, or an inhaler, as prescribed by your doctor, may be very helpful. You need to be sure that you understand which medications are preventive and which relieve symptoms.

Second, talk to your child to find out how he or she feels about exercise. Find out whether the child has been avoiding it, and if so, why. Then take steps to make exercise feel safe and possible for your child. This might involve finding some forms of exercise that your child is interested in, perhaps beginning with a family outing or a special adventure for you and your child alone. Take your child swimming, go on a hike together, kick a soccer ball around or shoot a few baskets—in short, find a way to get your child moving and active in a context where he or she can feel protected by you and safe from any possible embarrassment in front of friends.

Alternatively, your child may be chomping at the bit to exercise and/or to play with friends. It may be that your child will join in friends' games and sports contests as soon as he or she trusts that a breathing exercise or an inhaler will prevent or counter an asthma attack.

As with diet, finding the exercise habits that work for your child may take a bit of detective work on both your parts. It may also be that a solution that works for a while eventually stops working. Perhaps your child's friends love soccer for a while—and then switch to playing with dolls or video games, so that getting your child to exercise becomes a more private activity, less of a social event. Perhaps your child's friends love baseball, but your child feels most comfortable with swimming (the humid air at a swimming pool is especially soothing for people with asthma, although some react badly to either the chlorine in the water or the mold that tends to grow in damp places). Stay in touch and find ways to talk with your child about what he or she feels. With patience and creativity, you can find ways of exercise that your child will enjoy—and that will help keep him or her healthy.

## Working with Your Doctor

As in any doctor-patient relationship, your relationship with your child's doctor is a two-way street. You need information, advice, access to the latest thinking on medications, diet, exercise, and lifestyle. Your doctor needs information, too, as well as cooperation and respect. You both need a workable system for determining when and how you will contact your doctor in case of emergency, to report side effects of medication, or simply to get more information. You need a definite plan of action in case of an asthma attack.

*Developing Good Communication*   The key to your relationship with your child's doctor is communication. Follow the suggestions in Chapter 11 about how to get the most out of a doctor's visit—but supplement them by asking your doctor directly how he or she wants you to handle requests for information, problems, and emergencies. A nurse-educator may be your initial contact when you have a problem. If you have questions, concerns, or objections about what your doctor tells you, air your feelings.

Of course, doctors have busy lives and busy schedules, and parents of children with asthma often live with a great deal of stress and anxiety. The combination can make for frustration and misunderstanding on both sides. You should understand that your doctor may sometimes have a bad day, respond with impatience, or take a while to return a call. Your doctor should understand that you are legitimately worried about your child's health. Ideally, the two of you will work out a relationship that you can both live with.

*Keeping an Asthma Journal*   You can help your doctor follow your child's progress by keeping a daily journal, recording your child's symptoms, diet, encounters with allergy triggers, and responses to exercise, weather, and other environmental factors. Many physicians will have you keep a record of peak flows once or twice a day, depending on the severity of the disease. Here are some other items that you might note:

- *Symptoms.* Does your child suffer from coughing, wheezing, shortness of breath, runny or clogged nose, pallor, sleep problems, or fatigue?
- *Appearance.* Does the skin on your child's chest seem sucked in when your child tries to inhale? (Pay special attention to the skin between the ribs and above the collarbone.) This is called retraction and should prompt an immediate call to your physician.
- *Breathing habits.* Does your child take longer to breathe out than to breathe in? How fast is your child breathing? (Normal breathing is twenty-five to sixty breaths per minute for infants; twenty to thirty breaths per minute for children

under age four; fifteen to twenty-five breaths per minute for children aged five to fourteen; eleven to twenty-three breaths per minute for children aged fifteen to eighteen. Of course, when a person is asleep, his or her breathing is generally slower.)
- *Itching.* Does your child scratch under his or her chin or throat? (This kind of itchiness can indicate an asthmatic feeling.)

*Using a Peak-Flow Meter* Children over age six as well as adults can use this device, which measures the force with which a person exhales. Peak-flow meters allow a person with asthma another way to monitor his or her condition, as well as measure progress in response to a course of treatment.

Work with your doctor to make sure that both you and your child understand how your child should use the peak-flow meter. Then work with your child to keep a chart of peak-flow meter readings for you to share with your doctor. Children often enjoy making notations in a chart, especially if stars, stickers, or other playful items are involved. Older children may like the feeling that they have an important responsibility, such as gathering information for the doctor or keeping track of their progress with a new treatment.

Remember, too, that a peak-flow meter reading can be used to boost your child's confidence. If the meter shows normal-to-good lung functioning, your child can feel confident about engaging in exercise and play. By the same token, if the meter suggests a problem, you and your child can address it as soon as possible, before it becomes a debilitating attack.

Finally, be aware that peak-flow meter readings will naturally vary depending on the time of day. Whenever possible, take readings at the same time each day. Talk with your doctor about what variations you might expect, as well as to find out what he or she wants you to do in the event of a bad reading.

Also remember that the peak flow is effort-dependent—that is, it varies somewhat with the degree of effort. A child fearful of some event at school might consciously or subconsciously not blow as hard as he or she is capable of.

Moreover, the peak flow only measures large airway flow. It is possible to have worsening disease while still having a usual peak flow. Look at your other signs of distress and trust your judgment in deciding when to call your doctor.

## *Finding the Right Medications for Your Child*

The basic information in Chapter 12 will help you understand the asthma medications currently available to your child. Here are a few more specific points to help you work with your doctor to choose a treatment:

- Possible side effects of regular use of oral steroids are weight gain, immune suppression, thinning bones, growth suppression, and cataracts. Steroids are the most potent anti-inflammatory drugs and are used for severe attacks. They may also be needed regularly by the children with the most severe asthma. The inhaled steroids, if used correctly (with a spacer, and being sure to rinse the mouth afterward) are much less likely to cause any side effects.
- One type of leukotriene modifier, Singular, is available in a chewable tablet.
- Theophylline is used much less often. With higher doses, many children feel agitated and show symptoms that resemble hyperactivity when they are taking theophylline. Blood levels have to be monitored and are affected fever, diet, and many other medications. A low dose of theophylline may work together with other preventive medications to reduce symptoms without causing significant side effects.
- Children too young to use an inhaler can use a nebulizer, a machine that turns liquid medication into a fine mist. Nebulizers allow children (and adults) to absorb medication more slowly, at a controlled pace. Nebulizers are useful for any patient whose asthma is not well controlled with oral medications and inhalers. Both quick relief and long-term control medications can be administered by this route.

## The Emotional Side of Childhood Asthma

As pointed out throughout this book, having asthma is not just a physical experience. It also profoundly involves the mind and the emotions. This is especially true for a child with asthma—and for that child's family.

*"Who Am I When I'm Not Sick?"* From a child's point of view, it's difficult to separate "self" from sickness. A child's experience of himself or herself is often bound up with being sick, having been sick, or being afraid of getting sick. Likewise, it may be difficult for parents of children with asthma not to treat them as though their sickness were the most significant thing about them— a condition to be evoked every time decisions are made about what they can eat, where they can play, what they can do, when they go to bed. It can be quite a challenge, on the one hand, to realistically consider and care for the child's special health needs while, on the other hand, seeing him or her as a *whole* child, a child who occasionally needs to cut loose, to have special treats, to make mistakes, even to be "bad." If the child's asthma becomes the shadow always present with any bad behavior ("How could you sneak those extra cookies before dinner? Don't you know you have to be careful about your diet?"), let alone any good behavior ("It's nice you want to help with the housework, but there's too much dust for you—you might get sick"), everyone in the family, including the child, will start to see the sickness as synonymous with the child.

What's the solution? How can parents—let alone the child and his or her siblings—take realistic account of a chronic illness while still relating to the child as a human being? The answer begins with becoming aware of your feelings—and then sharing them.

### *How Do You Feel?*

Here are some of the feelings and experiences that we have found among parents of children with asthma:

- I know I'm being the typical overprotective parent—but I can't help it.

- Sometimes I get angry that my child needs so much attention.
- My child is just different from other children, and there's nothing we can do about it.
- My child is frustrated because of all the things she can't do—and I don't know how to help her.
- My child is always anxious, overly cautious, and avoids any kind of new experience or physical activity.
- I wish that—instead of my child—I could be the one to have asthma.
- I wish that I could breathe for my child when he has an attack.
- I miss so much sleep (or days at work, or something else) because of my child's asthma.
- I worry all the time that I'm not doing the right thing for my child.
- My child won't follow any of the rules about her asthma, and she ignores her condition—until she has an attack.
- My spouse is angry because I spend so much time with my child who has asthma.
- My child's siblings are angry because the child with asthma gets so much attention.
- I feel guilty because the asthma comes from my side of the family.
- I feel angry at my spouse because the asthma comes from his/her side of the family.
- My child "uses" asthma to get attention.
- I'm so worried about the long-term effects of medication—but I can't deny the medication to my child.
- I feel I could be doing more, somehow.
- This whole situation just makes me so sad for all of us—myself, my spouse, my other children, and my sick child.

*Separating Feelings and Actions* It's important to remember that there's a difference between feelings and actions. Knowing that sometimes you get angry even when it isn't "fair," that you sometimes wish you could just run away to a problem-free life (even though you'd never actually go), that you sometimes (or often) don't like being wakened in the middle of the night (even though, of course, you want to be with your sick child)—knowing and accepting these feelings in yourself can be remarkably liberating. If you can see that every parent, and particularly every parent of a child with asthma, has some of these feelings, you can begin to feel better about who you are and all that you do provide for your family and your child.

*Finding Support* If at all possible, join a support group for parents of children with asthma. Sometimes, just knowing that you're not alone can be an enormous comfort. Some parents also find that counseling of some kind helps them cope with the huge demands of having a child with asthma. A safe place to blow off steam, to explore difficult problems, to share troubling feelings, either with one's spouse or in privacy, can be a source of sustenance. Talking with a religious leader or a trusted friend or relative can also help you both to become aware of your feelings and to cope with them. These are resources that every parent needs from time to time, but the need can be especially urgent if they have a child with asthma.

*Time for "Time Out"* Finally, keeping a journal, meditating, or finding some way to take at least fifteen minutes out of your day, or an hour out of your week, as time for "just you," can also be a source of strength. Perhaps you and your spouse can work together to ensure that each of you gets just a little "time off" each week. If you're a single parent, perhaps you can find a friend or relative who'll take over for even a short time, so that you have a chance to recharge your batteries and reconnect to your own needs and interests. Having a child with asthma requires putting someone else's needs first a great deal of the time. Respect that work by giving yourself the support you need to do it.

### Sharing Feelings at Home

What happens after you get in touch with your own feelings and begin to accept them? The next step is to create a space within the family where both the child with asthma and the other family members can share their feelings, so that problems can be worked through together, rather than resented separately.

Many families find it helpful to start this process by having one or more sessions with a family counselor. This type of therapist is skilled at finding ways that each family member—from the child barely able to talk, to the middle siblings, to the parents—can express his or her feelings while becoming aware of the feelings of other family members. A good family counselor will also suggest ways that your whole family can continue to communicate, perhaps through family meetings, perhaps through making time for one-on-one communication among yourselves.

*Family Counseling* The basic principle of family counseling is that anything that affects one family member affects the whole family. A child's asthma certainly affects brothers, sisters, and parents. For example, having to find a new home for the family pet because it's making one child sick is a highly charged emotional issue. If your child with asthma is allergic to the pet, you have little choice about your action: let's assume that regardless of how anyone else feels about it, the pet must go. But if a child's brothers and sisters have room to say how angry, sad, or frustrated they feel about losing their beloved pet, if the child with asthma has room to say that he or she feels guilty, frightened, resentful, or sad as well, it's possible for these feelings to be worked through and resolved.

In some situations, family counseling—or family meetings without a counselor—can help raise solutions to a problem that you may not have thought of. ("What if we gave our pet to Aunt Jane and Uncle Thomas—then at least we could visit him!") In other cases, a family meeting might just air issues that help people understand each other better. ("Lucy, I had no idea you were so upset. I know this is a hard situation. I'm sorry—I'm upset, too.") Either way, making the space to acknowledge difficulties and involving everyone in coping with them can take a great deal of the pressure off you, the parent, leaving you free to focus your time and energy on the things that only you can do.

## Negotiating at School

One of your major responsibilities, as the parent of a child with asthma, is to negotiate with your child's school. Missed school days, rules about having asthma medication remain with the nurse, and the more amorphous question of how your child is treated are all major issues for parents of children with asthma. Here are some specific suggestions:

1. Recall that Section 504 of the Federal Rehabilitation Act entitles all students with chronic illness–including asthma–to health services and to any necessary changes in educational services. In other words, if your child is missing school because of asthma, he or she has a right to a workable plan for how to cope with the problem– and a right not to be penalized for illness. He or she also has a right not to be penalized for missing gym classes for medical reasons.

2. Keep the lines of communication open. Work with your child's teacher and the school's principal, nurse, and other staff to develop an asthma-management plan that applies to school life. You can contribute a list of your child's asthma triggers; the symptoms of an asthma attack; instructions on how to respond to certain symptoms or to certain peak-flow meter readings; information about your child's medications and possible side effects; and instructions on whom to contact in case of an emergency. You can find out from school personnel what their concerns are regarding schoolwork, gym classes, medical care, homework, and relationships with other children.

3. If your school does not allow any child to carry his or her own medications, and if you feel that your child needs immediate access to his or her asthma medication, discuss this concern as well. The law requires schools to provide medical support for children with asthma. If your–or your doctor's–definition of medical support includes your child carrying an inhaler, find a way to communicate this to the school.

4. As far as possible, involve your child in decisions about how to handle school matters. Children have strong feelings about receiving "special treatment" that makes them seem "different" from their peers. Of course, you, not your child, must have the last word on how to protect your child's health while ensuring him or her a good education. But again, your child may have solutions or suggestions you haven't yet thought of. Moreover, if your child is allowed to express his or her feelings and is involved actively in making plans work, you'll have a much happier family—and a much healthier child.

## *Ask Your Doctor ...*

- Have we correctly diagnosed my child's symptoms? Does he or she in fact have asthma? How do you know?
- Are there other tests we need to do to find out more about my child's allergies or asthma? What are they? How do they work? Why do you think we need them? What will we learn from them?
- How should we handle it when we have a question? When our child is having trouble? When there is an emergency?
- Can we come up with a written asthma-management plan, specifying what we should do in various situations: to prevent attacks; when an attack is occurring; in case of an emergency?
- Can we come up with a written asthma-management plan to present to our child's school, including information about asthma triggers, medication, symptoms, side effects, and emergency care?
- What foods should my child be avoiding?
- What kind of exercise can my child engage in?
- What can we do to make exercise as safe as possible for my child?
- What steps should we take to make our home as asthma-proof as possible?

- What else should we do to help my child avoid asthma/allergy triggers?
- What medications are safe for my child?
- What possible side effects will be caused by the medication you recommend? How should we respond to those side effects?
- What other alternatives are there for medication?
- In your experience of families with asthma, what issues should we be aware of? What advice do you have for us in coping with this situation?
- Can you recommend a family counselor, a parent support group, or other ways that we as a family can get support for this situation?

# Appendices

*Appendix A: Glossary of Terms Relating to Asthma*

*Appendix B: Food Groups*

*Appendix C: Medications and Asthma*

*Appendix D: National Organizations Dealing with Asthma and Lung-Related Disorders*

*Appendix E: National Treatment Centers (Adult and Pediatric)*

*Appendix F: Allergy Supplies*

*Appendix G: Bibliography*

# Appendix A

# Glossary of Terms Relating to Asthma

**acaracide**  Agent that kills dust mites.
**acetylcholine**  Chemical substance stored in nerve endings of parasympathetic nervous system released when nerves are stimulated, producing a response.
**adrenaline**  Trade name for epinephrine, the natural product of the adrenal gland; used to treat acute asthma and allergy reactions.
**adrenergic**  Name given to drugs derived from epinephrine, or to adrenalinelike drugs.
**aerosol**  Drug that can be sprayed or inhaled into the nose or lung.
**air sacs**  Common name for alveoli.
**airways**  Common name for bronchial tubes, or bronchi.
**airway hyperactivity**  The restriction or contraction of the bronchial tubes in response to substances or stimuli that occurs in asthmatics.
**allergen**  A substance that produces an allergic reaction.
**allergy**  A hypersensitive response to a normally harmless substance.
**alveoli**  Small air sacs in the lung where the exchange of oxygen and carbon dioxide takes place.
**anaphylaxis**  Medical term for the rapid onset of an extreme allergic reaction that can result in collapse, shock, or death.
**antibody**  A protein produced by the immune system that reacts with an antigen or an allergen.

**antigen** A substance that causes an antibody response in the body. The response may be protective (for example, the antibodies might cause allergic reactions).

**antihistamine** A type of drug used to reduce the effects of histamine in the treatment of allergies.

**atelectasis** A condition of the lungs, in which the alveoli collapse.

**atopy** Allergy or allergic sensitization.

**autonomic nervous system** The involuntary control system of the body that regulates blood pressure, pulse rate, and bronchial muscle tone.

**beta-agonist** Adrenalinelike medication that causes dilation of the bronchial tubes.

**beta blockade** The theory that attributes asthma to blocked or damaged beta receptors.

**beta receptors** Nerve endings that regulate bronchial tube condition.

**bronchial tubes** Air passages in and out of the lung.

**bronchioles** Tiny air passages that branch off from the bronchi.

**bronchiectasis** Abnormal dilation of the bronchus that causes considerable mucus secretion.

**bronchitis** Inflammation of the bronchial tubes.

**bronchoconstriction** Narrowing or closing of the bronchial tubes.

**bronchodilator** Medication that relaxes bronchial muscle and, in turn, dilates (opens or widens) the bronchial tubes.

**bronchospasm** Tightening or closure of airways.

**capillaries** Tiny blood vessels that collect oxygen in the lungs.

**carbon dioxide** Waste gas removed from the body via the lungs in exhaled air as a normal part of metabolism.

**chronic obstructive pulmonary disease (COPD)** Disease that results in diminished lung function; for example, emphysema, chronic bronchitis.

**cholinergic** Medication that stimulates the parasympathetic nervous system, leading to contraction of bronchial muscle in the lungs.

# Glossary of Terms Relating to Asthma

**cilia**  Tiny waving hairlike structures that remove debris from the lungs and carry it into the windpipe where it can be coughed up.

**corticosteroid**  Hormones produced by the cortex of the adrenal glands; also, artificial hormones used as anti-inflammatories in the treatment of asthma and other diseases.

**cromolyn sodium**  Important drug used in the treatment of asthma to prevent bronchospasm.

**cystic fibrosis**  Hereditary severe lung disease affecting children; can cause asthmalike symptoms.

**DPI**  Abbreviation for a Dry Powder Inhaler.

**dyspnea**  Shortness of breath.

**edema**  Accumulation of excess fluid in body tissues, causing swelling and weight gain.

**emphysema**  A chronic lung disease in which the walls of the alveoli become distended and the bronchial tubes are weakened.

**epiglottis**  Structure at the top of the larynx that prevents food and water from entering the trachea.

**extrinsic asthma**  Term used when exposure to an allergen is suspected of triggering asthma.

**FDA**  Abbreviation for the Food and Drug Administration, the federal agency charged with testing and approving medications.

**FEV**  Forced expiratory volume in one second; amount of air expelled in one second after a big breath.

**FVC**  Forced vital capacity; amount of air that can be expelled after a big breath.

**fungi**  Mold or mildew whose spores can trigger an asthmatic reaction.

**gas exchange**  Process by which the blood, as it flows through the lungs, absorbs oxygen and removes carbon dioxide.

**generic**  Name for drugs that do not carry a brand name; generic drugs are often less expensive than brand-name medications.

**glottis**  The elongated space between the vocal cords.

**hay fever**  A popular term for allergic reactions of the mucous membranes of the nose and upper respiratory passages.

**HEPA filter**  High-efficiency particulate air purifier. HEPA filters can be used in central ventilation systems, room air purifiers, and vacuum cleaners.

**histamine**  A chemical substance normally present in the body that is released when tissues are injured or an allergic reaction occurs.

**humidification**  The addition of moisture to the air.

**hyperreactive airways**  Airways that become sensitive, irritated, or tight when exposed to normally harmless substances; also called hyperactive, hypersensitive.

**hyperventilation**  An increase in inspiration or expiration as a result of deeper and/or faster breathing; can cause anxiety, dizziness, and fainting, among other symptoms.

**hypoventilation**  The reduced rate and depth of respiration.

**hypoxia**  The absence of adequate oxygen in body tissues.

**immune system**  The defense mechanisms of the body that protect against invasion of diseases and foreign substances. Dysregulation of the immune system leads to the development of allergic conditions (asthma and hay fever) or allergic reactions to food and drugs.

**immunoglobulin E**  The specific antibody produced by the immune system that leads to allergic reactions; also known as IgE.

**immunotherapy**  Allergy treatments in which small amounts of an allergen are injected into the body to lead to less reactivity; also known as "desensitization" or "allergy shots."

**inflammatory cascade**  A chain of chemical reactions that produce inflammation.

**inhalation therapy**  The administration of drugs or vapors to the lungs by breathing in.

**intradermal skin test**  The injection of a fluid substance under the skin to test for hypersensitivity.

**intravenous** The injection of a drug or solution into the veins.

**intrinsic asthma** Refers to a kind of asthma associated with other respiratory conditions, such as sinusitis or bronchitis, and in which allergy triggers are not identified.

**larynx** The modified upper part of the trachea that contains the vocal cords.

**lymphocytes** White blood cells that govern the immune system. They are classified as T-cells, B-cells, and natural killer cells.

**mast cells** Found in connective tissue, skin, and mucosa, including that of the bronchial tubes, mast cells contain histamine and other substances that are instrumental in an allergic reaction.

**medulla** The part of the lower brain that controls respiration, coughing, swallowing, and other metabolic functions.

**mixed asthma** A combination of extrinsic and intrinsic asthma.

**mucus** Slippery fluid secreted by mucous membranes that line the bronchial tubes; often called phlegm or sputum. Important in cleaning foreign particles from the lungs.

**nebulizer** An atomizer or sprayer that creates a fine mist that can be inhaled into the lungs.

**neutrophil** A type of white blood cell that is often involved in immune reactions.

**particulates** Fine, airborne soot; a component of air pollution produced by fuel combustion.

**peak-flow meter** A portable device that measures air flow as it is expelled from the lungs.

**pharynx** The upper portion of the throat; it is the passageway for air from the nose to the larynx and for food from the mouth to the esophagus.

**pleura** The membrane that covers the lungs.

**pleurisy** An inflammation of the pleura.

**pollen** Plant parts released by trees, grasses, and weeds that act as allergens in the body.

**prednisone** A steroid drug, similar to cortisone, that is often used to treat an asthma relapse.

**prick test** Skin test in which a drop of allergen is placed on the skin and then the skin is pricked with a needle.

**prn** Medical abbreviation for "take as needed."

**pulmonary function tests** Breathing tests that indicate how well the lungs are moving air.

**rales** Refers to an abnormal sound heard in lungs that is produced when air passes through a narrowed passage or one that contains moisture.

**RAST** Abbreviation for radioallergosorbent test, a blood test that can identify allergies to specific substances.

**scratch test** A test for allergies in which the skin is lightly scratched and a drop of allergen is placed on the scratched area.

**spirometer** A device that tests airflow when the patient breathes.

**sputum** The fluid substance brought up by coughing or clearing one's throat.

**tachypnea** Rapid breathing.

**theophylline** Refers to drugs in the xanthine family that relax bronchial passages and stimulate the central nervous system.

**trachea** The large airway connecting the mouth to the bronchial tubes; also known as the windpipe.

**triggers** Conditions or substances that cause asthma attacks.

**urticaria** The eruption of hives; usually represents a systemic allergic response.

**wheezing** Blowing or whistling sounds produced by airway narrowing, typical of asthma.

# Appendix B
# Food Groups

The following is a list of food groups. If you develop asthmatic symptoms as a result of eating one food in a specific group or family, you *might* be somewhat more likely to become sensitive to other foods in that group.

**Animal Groups**

*Amphibians:* frog

*Birds (flesh and organs):* chicken, Cornish hen, duck, goose, grouse, guinea hen (fowl), partridge, pheasant, pigeon, quail, squab, turkey

*Crustaceans:* crab, crayfish, lobster, prawn, shrimp

*Eggs (bird):* white, whole, yolk

*Fish (representative families)*
Acipenseridae: sturgeon (caviar)
Anguillidae: eel
Argentidae: smelt
Carangidae: pompano
Centrarchidae: black bass, crappie, sunfish
Clupidae: herring, sardine, shad, sprat
Cyprinidae: carp
Esodidae: muscallonge, pickerel, pike
Gadidae: cod, haddock, hake, pollack, scrod
Mugillidae: mullet
Percidae: perch
Pleuronectidae: flounder, halibut
Salmonidae: grayling, salmon, trout, whitefish

Scienidae: bonito, mackerel, tuna
Serranidae: grouper, rockfish, white bass
Siluridae: bullhead, catfish
Soleidae: sole
Sparidae: porgy, red snapper
Stolephoridae: anchovy
Xyphidae: swordfish

*Red Meats (flesh and internal organs)*

1. Bovidae
   Cow: beef, calf, steer, veal
   Gelatin
   Goat
   Ox
   Sheep: lamb, mutton, sweetbread
2. Suidae (pig): bacon, boar, ham, hog, pig, pork, sausage, scrapple, sow, swine

*Milk Products (cow, goat)*

butter
buttermilk
casein
cheese
cream: sour, whipped, ice cream, lactalbumin
milk: condensed, evaporated, homogenized, powdered, raw, skimmed, selected infant formulas
yogurt

***Mollusks:*** abalone, clam, cockle, mussel, octopus, oyster, quahog, scallop, snail (escargot), squid

***Reptiles:*** alligator, crocodile, rattlesnake, terrapin, turtle

## Plant Groups

***Apple Family:*** apple, cider, vinegar (apple cider), crab apple, loquat, pear, quince, quince seed

***Banana Family:*** banana, plantain

*Beech Family:* beechnut, chestnut, chinquapin

*Birch Family:* filbert (hazelnut), wintergreen (*Betula* spp.)

*Buckwheat Family:* buckwheat, rhubarb, sorrel

*Cashew Family:* cashew, mango, pistachio

*Citrus Family:* citron, grapefruit, kumquat, lemon, lime, orange, tangelo, tangerine

*Cola Nut Family:* chocolate (cacao), cocoa, cocoa butter; cola (kola) nut

*Fungi:*

mushroom

truffle

yeast: baker's, brewer's, distiller's, Fleischmann's, lactose fermenting, lager beer

*Ginger Family:* cardomom (cardomon, cardamum), east India arrowroot, ginger, turmeric

*Goosefoot Family:* beet, lamb's quarters, spinach, Swiss chard

*Gourd (melon) Family:* cantaloupe (muskmelon), casaba (winter muskmelon), Chinese watermelon, citron melon, cucumber, gherkin, honeydew melon, Persian melon, pumpkin, summer squash, watermelon, winter squash

*Grape Family:* champagne, grape, raisin, vinegar (wine), wine (grape)

*Grass (cereal) Family:* bamboo, barley, corn (maize), hominy, malt (germinated grain), millet, oat, popcorn, rice, rye, sorghum, sugar cane; wheat: bran, germ, gliadin, globulin, glutenin, leucosin, proteose

*Heath Family:* black huckleberry, blueberry, cranberry, wintergreen (*Pyrola* spp.)

*Laurel Family:* avocado, bay leaf, cinnamon, sassafras

*Lecythis Family:* Brazil nut

*Lily Family:* aloe, asparagus, chives, garlic, onion, sarsaparilla, shallot

*Madder Family:* coffee

*Mallow Family:* cottonseed, marshmallow, okra (gumbo)

*Mint Family:* balm, basil, catnip, horehound, Japanese artichoke, lavender, marjoram, mint, oregano, peppermint, rosemary, sage, savory, spearmint, thyme

*Morning Glory Family:* sweet potato, yam

*Mustard Family:* broccoli, brussels sprouts, cabbage, cauliflower, collards, garden cress, horseradish, kale, kohlrabi, mustard, rutabaga, turnip, watercress

*Myrtle Family:* allspice, clove, guava, myrtle, pimento

*Nightshade Family:* bell pepper, cayenne pepper, chili (paprika) (red pepper), eggplant, ground cherry, melon pear, potato (white), strawberry tomato, tobacco, tomato, tree tomato

*Nutmeg Family:* mace, nutmeg

*Olive Family:* jasmine, olive

*Orchid Family:* vanilla

*Palm Family:* cabbage palm, coconut, date, heart of palm

*Papaya Family:* papain, papaya

*Parsley Family:* anise, carrot, celeriac, celery, coriander, dill, fennel, parsley, parsnip

*Pea (legume) Family:* acacia, alfalfa, black-eyed pea (cowpea), broad bean (fava bean), carob bean (St John's bread), chick pea (garbanzo), common bean, kidney, navy, pinto, string (green), jack bean, lentil, licorice, lima bean, mesquite, peanut, soybean, tamarind, tragacanth

*Pepper Family:* black pepper

*Pine Family:* juniper, pine nut (pignolia)

*Pineapple Family:* pineapple

*Plum Family:* almond, apricot, cherry, nectarine, peach, plum, prune

*Poppy Family:* poppyseed

*Rose Family:* black raspberry, blackberry, boysenberry, dewberry, loganberry, red raspberry, strawberry

*Saxifrage Family:* currant, gooseberry

*Sunflower Family:* absinthe (sagebrush, wormwood), artichoke, camomile, chicory, dandelion, endive, escarole, Jerusalem artichoke, lettuce, oyster plant (salsify), safflower, sunflower seed, tansy, tarragon

*Tea Family*

*Walnut Family:* black walnut, butternut, English walnut, hickory nut, pecan

## Sources of Salicylate

*Foods ("Natural" salicylates that may or may not cause symptoms in aspirin-sensitive people)*

| | |
|---|---|
| *Beverages:* | tea, root beer, birch beer |
| *Meat:* | corned beef, meat processed with vinegar |
| *Fat:* | salad dressing, mayonnaise, avocado, olives |
| *Starch:* | white potatoes, products with potato starch |
| *Vegetables:* | cucumbers, green pepper and other peppers, tomatoes |
| *Fruits:* | apples, apple cider, apricots, blackberries, boysenberries, cherries, currants, dewberries, gooseberries, huckleberries, maraschino cherries, grapes, melon, nectarines, peaches, raisins, raspberries, prunes, plums |
| *Sweets/desserts:* | any mint or wintergreen product |
| *Miscellaneous:* | cloves, pickles, catsup, tartar sauce, tabasco sauce, cider vinegar, beer, wine, distilled alcoholic beverages (except vodka) |

### Drugs

| | | |
|---|---|---|
| Acetidine | Bufferin | Liquiprin |
| Alka-Seltzer | Coricidin | Midol |
| Anacin | Darvon compound | Pepto-Bismol |
| Anahist | Dristan | Persistin |
| A.C.P. | Ecotrin | Sal-Sayne |
| aspirin | Empirin compound | Stanback |
| BC | Excedrin | Theracin |
| Bromo-Quinine | 4-Way Cold capsules | Trigesic |
| Bromo-Seltzer | Inhiston | |

### Flavoring

| | | |
|---|---|---|
| antiseptics | gum | oil of wintergreen |
| breath sweeteners | lozenges | perfumes |
| candies (some) | mouth wash | toothpaste |

# Appendix C
# Medications and Asthma

*How to Use a Nebulizer with Y-Tube (Air Compressor–Driven)*

1. Follow instructions given by your physician for preparing the solution.
2. Remove plastic plugs and add extender.
3. Check the nebulizer by putting your finger over the Y-tube to see that a mist comes out of the mouthpiece.
4. Blow out a little air beyond the normal expiration.
5. Put the mouthpiece into your mouth and close your lips around it.
6. Put your finger over the Y-tube.
7. Take in a very slow maximum breath, as if you were sipping hot soup, while keeping your finger over the Y-tube.
8. When you can get no more air or medicine into your lungs, take your finger off the Y-tube.
9. Take the mouthpiece out of your mouth, let the air out, breathe normally for one minute, and check for the indicators of sufficient medicine.

*How to Use a Nebulizer without a Y-Tube*

1. Follow instructions given by your physician for preparing the solution.
2. Remove plastic plugs and add extender.
3. Turn on and place the mask over your face or the mouthpiece in your mouth. (Some infants are frightened by the apparatus, and will get some medication if the outflow is held in front of their nose or mouth.)

4. Breathe normally.
5. When the medication is used up, clean as directed.

## *How to Clean Your Nebulizer*

To prevent lung infection from a dirty nebulizer, use the following simple cleaning methods.

### *Before Each Treatment:*

1. Use a clean eyedropper or syringe to measure medications unless it is provided in a unit dose that simply has to be opened. Be careful not to touch the tip—you may contaminate it.
2. Replace bottle caps promptly and close tightly.

### *After Each Treatment:*

1. Rinse nebulizer under a strong stream of warm water for thirty seconds.
2. Shake off excess moisture. Allow to air-dry on a clean towel. Before storing your equipment, you may want to dry the nebulizer by attaching it to your air compressor (if you have one) and blowing it dry.

### *Monday-Wednesday-Friday or Every Other Day*

1. Wash plastic nebulizer completely with a mild dish soap and warm water. Never immerse the compressor (motor).
2. Rinse thoroughly under running, warm tap water.
3. Completely immerse nebulizer and tubing for thirty minutes in a solution of one part white vinegar and two parts water. Discard vinegar solution after each use.
4. Rinse nebulizer thoroughly under running, warm tap water for one minute.
5. Allow to air-dry on a clean towel.
6. Keep the nebulizer and eyedropper (or syringe) clean and dry. Store in a closed plastic bag.
7. Clean canister-type inhalers in the same manner.

## Commonly Prescribed Beta-2 Agonists

| Generic Name | Brand Name | Method | Length of Action |
|---|---|---|---|
| Epinephrine | Adrenalin | subcutaneous injection | very short-acting–up to 15–20 minutes |
| | Sus-Phrine | subcutaneous injection | longer-acting–2–4 hours |
| Isoetharine | Bronkometer | metered-dose inhaler | 4–8 hours |
| | Bronkosol | solution for nebulizer | 4–8 hours; CAUTION: contains sulfites |
| Metaproterenol | Alupent, Metaprel | metered-dose inhaler | 3–5 hours |
| | | solution for nebulizer | 3–5 hours |
| | | tablets or syrup | up to 4 hours |
| | | long-acting tablets | 12 hours |
| Albuterol | Proventil, Ventolin | metered-dose inhaler | 4–6 hours |
| | | tablets | 4–6 hours |
| Terbutaline | Brethine, Bricanyl | subcutaneous injection | 4–6 hours |
| | | metered-dose inhaler | 4–6 hours |
| | | tablets | 4–6 hours |
| Pirbuterol | Matair | breath-activated inhaler | 4–7 hours |
| Salmeterol | Severent | metered-dose inhaler | 12 hours. CAUTION: *Never* use more than twice a day, or for an acute attack! |

*Medications:*

cimetidine (Tagamet)

allopurinol (Zyloprim)

erythromycin (Erythrocin and others)

troleandomycin (Tao)

propranolol (Inderal)

methyldopa (Aldomet)

oral contraceptives

trivalent influenza vaccine

Other drugs that have an adverse effect on the liver, such as certain cancer chemotherapy agents

*May Decrease Theophylline Levels:*

Diet high in protein and low in carbohydrates

Cigarette or marijuana use

*Medications:*

barbiturates (e.g., phenobarbital)

carbamazepine (Tegretol)

phenytoin (Dilantin)

rifampin

## Side Effects of Steroid Drugs and How to Minimize Them

The following is only a partial list of possible adverse reactions, focusing on ones that may be at least partially controlled by the patient. Keep in mind that many of these are reversible once the medication can be stopped.

### Skin

*Acne:* Cleanse skin thoroughly but gently with mild soap.

*Tendency to bruise, thinning of skin:* Avoid abrasive or irritating materials. Use care when walking or running.

### Gastrointestinal System

*Risk of ulcers:* Take drugs with food to minimize gastric irritation. Use antacids or other antiulcer medication as prescribed. Report signs of abdominal pain or bleeding, including dark, tarry stools, to physician.

*Weight gain:* Watch food intake to minimize increased weight. Emphasize low-calorie, high-fiber foods that satisfy increased appetite. Report increases of five or more pounds to physician. Certain steroids promote sodium and water retention more than others and may result in weight gain and swelling of ankles and feet.

### Hormonal

*Osteoporosis:* People at high risk should have regular measurements of bone density to avoid excess thinning and risk of fracture. Vitamin D and calcium supplements and a regular exercise program help prevent steroid-induced bone loss. Postmenopausal women should consider estrogen replacement based on discussions with their gynecologist or primary physician.

*Diabetes:* Patients with latent or current diabetes may become hyperglycemic and require increased doses of insulin or oral hypoglycemics. Dietary control of weight gain is important.

### Metabolic

*Potassium deficiency:* Add an oral supplement or good sources of potassium to diet (leafy green vegetables, whole grains, citrus fruit, and bananas). Report signs of deficiency (muscle twitching, spasm, or cramps) to your doctor.

*Calcium deficiency:* Include diary products in diet and report signs of deficiency (muscle twitching, spasm, or cramps) to physician.

### Eyes

*Cataracts, increased risk:* Report any vision changes promptly to physician. Patients who do not have symptoms should have a vision exam every six to twelve months, including slit lamp and tonometry (internal pressure) check.

### Immune System

*Increased risk of infection:* See physician for infections that persist in spite of measures normally taken to combat them. If the patient is exposed to chicken pox and has not had it or the vaccine, the physician should be notified immediately.

# Appendix D

# National Organizations Dealing with Asthma and Lung-Related Disorders

**National Groups**

Action on Smoking and Health (ASH)
2013 H St. N.W.
Washington, D.C. 20006
202-659-4310
http://www.ash.org

Allergy and Asthma Network
Mothers of Asthmatics, Inc.
3554 Chain Bridge Rd.
(Suite 200)
Fairfax, VA 22030
1-800-878-4403
http://www.podi.com/health/aanma

Allergy Information Association
65 Tromley Dr.
Etobicoke, Ontario M9B 5Y7
Canada

American Academy of Allergy, Asthma, and Immunology
611 East Wells St.
Milwaukee, WI 53202
1-800-822-2762
http://www.AAAI.org

American Association for Respiratory Care
11030 Ables Lane
Dallas, TX 75229-4593
972-243-2272
http://www.AARC.org

American College of Allergy, Asthma, and Immunology
85 West Algonquin Rd.
(Suite 550)
Arlington Heights, IL 60005
1-800-842-7777
847-427-1200
http://www.allergy.mcg.edu

# National Organizations Dealing with Asthma

American Lung Association
1740 Broadway
New York, NY 10010
212-315-8700
http://www.lungusa.org

Asthma and Allergy
  Foundation (AAFA)
1125 15th St. N.W. (Suite 502)
Washington, DC 20005
1-800-7-ASTHMA
202-466-7643
http://www.aafa.org

Asthma Control Institute
  from Glaxo-Wellcome
5 Moore Dr.
Research Triangle, NC 27709
1-800-843-2474

Asthma Foundation
  of Southern Arizona
P.O. Box 30069
Tucson, AZ 85751-0069
520-323-6046

The Food Allergy Network
10400 Eaton Pl. (Suite 107)
Fairfax, VA 22030-2208
1-800-929-4040
703-691-3179
http://www.foodallergy.org

National Institute of Allergy
  and Infectious Diseases
  (NIAID)
9000 Rockville Pike
Bethesda, MD 20205
301-496-5717
http://www.niaid.nih.gov

National Jewish Medical
  and Research Center
1400 Jackson St.
Denver, CO 80206
1-800-222-LUNG (222-5864)
http://www.njc.org

Smoke Signal
P.O. Box 99688
San Francisco, CA 94109
415-776-3739

To find local or state organizations, contact the American Lung Association, American Cancer Society, or the American Heart Association. Many states and cities have chapters of GASP (Groups Against Smoking Pollution), and organizations devoted to enacting and enforcing laws protecting nonsmokers' rights.

## Help Lines

This service is staffed by specially trained nurses at the National Jewish Medical and Research Center in Denver, Colorado.
1-800-222-LUNG

The Asthma and Allergy Foundation's Headquarters in Washington, DC 1-800-7-ASTHMA: Asthma Information Line. Provides written material on asthma and allergies. Operates 24 hours a day.
1-800-822-ASTHMA

The toll-free physician referral service of the American College of Allergy, Asthma, and Immunology.
1-800-842-7777

The National Asthma Information Center administered by the National Heart, Lung, Blood Institutes (NHBLI).
1-301-951-3260

# Appendix E

# National Treatment Centers (Adult and Pediatric)

The Alfred I. Dupont Hospital
   for Children
Asthma Program
1600 Rockland Rd.
Wilmington, DE 19803
302-651-4000

Asthmatic Children's
   Foundation of New York
Residential Treatment Center
15 Spring Valley Rd.
Ossining, NY 10562
914-762-2110

Blythedale Children's Hospital
95 Broadhurst Ave.
Valhalla, NY 10595
914-592-7555

Brigham and Women's Hospital
75 Francis St.
Boston, MA 02115
617-732-1995

Children's Hospital
34th St. and Civic Blvd.
Philadelphia, PA 19104
215-590-1000

Children's Hospital
300 Longwood Ave.
Boston, MA 02115
617-735-7602

Children's Seashore
   House
35 South Annapolis
Atlantic City, NJ 08401
609-347-6157

Georgetown University School
   of Medicine
3800 Reservoir Rd. N.W.
Washington, DC 20007
202-887-8219

Health Hill Hospital for
   Children
2801 Martin Luther King
Cleveland, OH 44104
216-721-5400

Hospital for Sick
   Children
1731 Bunker Hill Rd.
Washington, DC 20017
202-832-4400

Institute for Asthma
 and Allergy
Washington Hospital
 Center
106 Irving St. N.W.
Washington, DC 20010
1-800-ASTHMA-5
202-877-7777

Johns Hopkins Asthma
 and Allergy Center
301 Bayview Blvd.
Baltimore, MD 21223
301-550-2101

La Rabida Children's
 Hospital
East 65th St. at Lake Michigan
Chicago, IL 60649
773-363-6700

Mayo Foundation
200 First St. Southwest
Rochester, MN 55905
507-284-2789

Medical College of Georgia
Allergy-Immunology Service
1125 15th St.
Augusta, GA 30912
706-721-2390

National Jewish Medical
 and Research Center
1400 Jackson St.
Denver, CO 80206
(303) 398-1656
1-800-423-8891

Northwestern University
 Medical School
303 East Chicago Ave.
Chicago, IL 60611
(312) 649-8172

Scripps Clinic and Research
 Foundation
10666 North Torrey Pines Rd.
La Jolla, CA 92037
(619) 457-8686

State University of New York
SUNY Health Sciences
 Center, T-16,
 Room 040
Stony Brook, NY 11794
(518) 444-2272

Tulane University School
 of Medicine
1700 Perdido Street
New Orleans, LA 70112
(504) 588-5578

University of Alabama
 University Station
Birmingham, AL 35294-3300
(205) 934-3370

University of Iowa Hospitals
 and Clinics
Iowa City, IA 52242
(319) 358-2117

University of Texas
Dept. of Medicine
 and Microbiology

UT Southwestern Medical
   Center
5324 Harry Hines Blvd.
Dallas, TX 75235-9048
(214) 888-2555

University of Virginia
Division of Allergy
   and Clinical
   Immunology
Health Services Center
Box 225
Charlottesville, VA 22908
(804) 924-5917

University of Washington
Dept. of Medicine, SJ-10
Seattle, WA 98195
(208) 543-3780

St. Mary's Hospital for
   Children
Bayside, NY 11376
(718) 990-8800

**Regional Resources
for Educational
Materials**

Allergy and Asthma
   Association of South
   Carolina
P.O. Box 23493
Columbia, SC 29224-3493

# Appendix F
# Allergy Supplies

Allergy Control Products, Inc.
96 Danbury Rd.
Ridgefield, CT 06877
1-800-422-DUST

American Breathing
  Association
6488 Fiesta Dr.
Dept. 300
Columbus, OH 43235-5201
1-800-735-4772

Bio-Tech Health Systems, Ltd.
P.O. Box 18398
Chicago, IL 60618
1-800-621-5545

Envirahealth Inc.
34 South Broadway
White Plains, NY 10601
1-800-877-7772

Environmental Health
  Shopper
P.O. Box 239
Fate, TX 75132
1-800-447-1100

National Allergy Supply, Inc.
4400 Abbotts Bridge Rd.
P.O. Box 1658
Duluth, GA 30096
1-800-522-1948

# Appendix G
# Bibliography

The following books can provide additional information about asthma.

Brisco, Paula. *Asthma: Questions You Have, Answers You Need*. Philadelphia: People's Medical Society, 1994.

Brookes, Tim. *Catching My Breath: An Asthmatic Explores His Illness*. New York: Random House, 1995.

Gershwin, Dr. M. Eric, and Dr. E. L. Klingelhofer. *Asthma: Stop Suffering Start Living, 2$^{nd}$ edition*. Reading, MA: Addison-Wesley, 1992.

Gordon Dr. Neil F. *Breathing Disorders: Your Complete Exercise Guide*. Champaign, IL: Human Kinetics Publishers, 1993.

Haas, Dr. Francois, and Dr. Sheila Sperber Haas. *The Chronic Bronchitis and Emphysema Handbook*. New York: John Wiley & Sons, 1990.

——. *The Essential Asthma Book: A Manual for Asthmatics of All Ages*. New York: Ballantine, 1987.

Hannaway, Dr. Paul J. *The Asthma Self-Help Book: How to Live a Normal Life in Spite of Your Condition*. Rocklin, CA: Prima Publishing, 1992.

Harrington, Geri. *The Asthma Self-Care Book*. New York: Harper Collins, 1991.

Hogshead, Nancy, and Gerald S. Couzens. *Asthma and Exercise*. New York: Henry Holt and Company, 1993.

Ridgway, Roy. *Asthma: A Comprehensive Guide to Gentle, Safe and Effective Treatment*. Rockport, MA: Element, Inc., 1994.

Sander, Nancy. *A Parent's Guide to Asthma: How You Can Help Your Child Control Asthma at Home, School, and Play*. New York: Penguin, 1994.

Weinstein, Dr. Allan M. *Asthma: The Complete Guide to Self-Management of Asthma and Allergies for Patients and Their Families*. New York: Ballantine, 1987.

# Index

## A

Acupuncture, alternative strategies, 143–144
Additives. *See* Food additives
Adult-onset asthma, 4, 35–37. *See also* Asthma; Childhood asthma
Aerobic exercise, 131
African Americans, asthma and, 42–43
Air conditioner, indoor environmental control, 93, 94
Air pollution. *See also* Workplace
  asthma and, 45–46
  environmental control, 106–108
  exercise and, 128
Alcoholic beverages, food allergy awareness, 77
Allergen identification, indoor environmental control, 90–92
Allergies, 60–72. *See also* Asthma; Food allergies
  asthma and, 13, 17–18, 37, 39
  asthma survey, 58
  atopy and, 61
  childhood asthma, environmental control, 181–184. *See also* Childhood asthma
  diagnosis of, 81–82
  doctor questions, 72
  downward spiral in, 62
  emotional and physical reactions, 63
  food allergy responses, 69–71. *See also* Food allergies
  food groups, listing of, 205–210
  immune system and, 65–68
  infections and, 68–69
  new, development of, 61–62
  supply sources for control of, 222
  symptoms of, 63–65, 71–72
  triggers of
    doctor questions, 83
    in foods, 73–79
    in medicines, 79–81
    synergy in, 108
Allergy shots, medication, 173–174
Allergy tests, described, 33
Alternative strategies, 140–148
  acupuncture, 143–144
  chiropractic, 145
  doctor questions, 147–148
  exploration of, 141–142
  herbal medicine, 142–143
  hypnosis, 145–147
  osteopathy, 144–145
  visualization process, 147
Anaphylactic reaction, food allergy responses, 69–70
Angiotensin converting enzyme inhibitors, allergy triggers, 81
Animal dander, indoor environmental control, 91, 92
Anticholinergics, bronchodilators, 166
Antihistamines:
  allergies and, 66
  medication, 173
Antihypertensive drugs, allergy triggers, 81

# INDEX

Anti-inflammatory drugs, 167–172
   cromolyn sodium and
      nedocromil, 171–172
   leukotriene modifiers, 172
   steroids, 167–171
Arterial Blood Gases (ABG) test,
      described, 32
Aspirin, allergy triggers, 79–80
Asthma. *See also* Allergies;
      Childhood asthma
   additives and, 47
   allergy and, 13, 17–18
   alternative strategies, 140–148.
      *See also* Alternative
      strategies
   causes of, 16–17, 44–48
   climate and, 10
   contagion, 9
   costs of, 44
   death rates, 14
   defined, 16
   diagnosis of, 29–34, 48–49
   doctor questions for, 39–40
   environmental factors, 13
   exercise and, 11
   facts about, 4–14
   food groups, listing of, 205–210
   genetics, 8–9
   glossary of terms, 199–204
   holistic approach and, vii–viii,
      50–59. *See also* Holistic
      approach
   industrialization and, 45–46,
      106–108
   intrinsic versus extrinsic, 7–8, 17
   lung damage, 11
   medical cure, 12
   medical profession and, 47–48
   national organizations, listed,
      216–221
   parents of children with, 49–50.
      *See also* Childhood asthma
   patterns of, 38
   poverty and, 42–43
   prevalence of, 41–44
   preventive measures, 13–14
   psychological profile, 12–13
   psychosomatic illness, 6–7
   risk factors, 9–10
   social relations and, 49
   stress, 7
   types of, 34–40
      adult-onset asthma, 35–37
      exercise-induced asthma, 35
      nocturnal asthma, 34–35
      seasonal asthma, 35
      variations in, 37–38
Asthma attack:
   components of, 27–29
   described, 24–25
   effects of, 26
   life threatening, 25–26
Asthma journal. *See* Journals
Atopy, allergies and, 61

## B

Beta-agonists:
   allergy triggers, 80–81
   bronchodilators, 159–163
   commonly prescribed, 213–215
Biofeedback, breathing exercise,
      132
Blood stream:
   allergy symptoms, 64
   IgE level tests, described, 82
Breathing:
   actions, 53
   environmental control, 85–86
   healthy process, 18–22
   inflammation and constriction,
      22–24
Breathing exercise, 131–139. *See also*
      Exercise
   biofeedback, 132
   described, 134–138
   hyperventilation, 131
   self-instruction, 132–133, 133–134
Bronchiolitis, defined, 180

Bronchitis, defined, 180
Bronchodilators, 159–166
   anticholinergics, 166
   beta-agonists, 159–163, 213–215
   epinephrine, 163
   theophylline, 164–166
Bronchoscopy, described, 34
Brookes, Tim, 51–52
Building-related illness, workplace, 104–105

## C

Carbon dioxide, indoor environmental control, 96–97, 98–99
Centers for Disease Control (CDC), 42
Chemicals, volatile, indoor environmental control, 97, 99
Chest inflation, asthma attack, 28–29
Chest pain, asthma attack, 28
Chest X ray, described, 33
Childhood asthma, 4, 176–197. *See also* Asthma
   adult asthma and, 7, 180–181
   diet and nutrition, 184–186
   doctor-patient relationship, 187–188
   doctor questions, 196–197
   effects of, 177–178
   emotional factors, 191–194
   environmental control, 181–184
   exercise, 186–187
   infections and, 69
   journals, 188–189
   medication, 190
   parents and, 49–50, 178
   peak-flow meter, 189–190
   prevalence of, 42, 43, 177
   psychological profile, 12–13
   schools and, 195–196
   warning signs of, 178–180
Chiropractic, alternative strategies, 145
Cigarette smoke:
   asthma risk factors, 10
   childhood asthma, environmental control, 182
   indoor environmental control, 95–96, 98
Cleaning products, indoor environmental control, 97, 99
Climate, asthma and, 10
Cockroaches, indoor environmental control, 91–92, 93
Complete Blood Count (CBC) test, described, 33
Conjunctivitis, allergy symptoms, 64
Constriction, breathing, 22–24
Contagion, asthma, 9
Cool-downs, exercise, 130, 131
Corticosteroids, anti-inflammatory drugs, 167–171
Cosmetics, indoor environmental control, 98
Costs, of asthma, 44
Cotton-dust asthma, 37
Coughing, asthma attack, 27–28
Couzens, Gerald S., 127
Cravings, allergies and, 71
Cromolyn sodium, anti-inflammatory drugs, 171–172
Croup, defined, 179
Cystic fibrosis, defined, 180

## D

Dander (animal), indoor environmental control, 91, 92
Death rates, asthma, 14, 41–42, 43
Dehumidifier, indoor environmental control, 93, 94
Dehydration, asthma attack, 29

# INDEX

Deodorants, indoor environmental control, 98
Diagnosis. *See also* Testing
 of allergies, 81–82
 of asthma, 29–34, 48–49
 of childhood asthma, 178–180
 doctor questions for, 39–40
Diaphragm, breathing exercise, 134–138
Diary. *See* Journals
Diet and nutrition:
 actions, 53
 asthma and, 47
 childhood asthma, 184–186
 doctors and, 123–124, 153
 food allergy awareness, 73–79
 food groups, listing of, 205–210
 holistic approach, 118–123
 steroids, 170–171
Diffusing capacity test, described, 32
Doctors, 149–156
 changing of, 155–156
 childhood asthma, 187–188
 communication with, 150–151
 medication, 158
 office visits, 151–153
 peak-flow meter, 153–155
 relationship with, questions for, 58–59, 156
 working with, 53–55
Drug interactions, theophylline, 165–166. *See also* Medication
Dust mites, indoor environmental control, 91, 92–93

## E

Elimination diet, food allergy awareness, 75–77
Emotional factors:
 breathing exercise, 137–138
 childhood asthma, 191–194
 holistic approach and, 111–112, 114–116

Emphysematous asthma, 37
Engler, Renata, 141, 142, 143
Environmental control, 53, 84–100
 air pollution, 106–108
 asthma, 13
 breathing, 85–86
 childhood asthma, 181–184
 coping with, 99
 doctor questions, 100, 108
 indoors, 89–99
  actions, 92–94
  allergen identification, 90–92
  irritants, 95–99
 outdoors, 86–89
  molds, 88–89
  pollens, 86–88
 supply sources for, 222
 workplace, 101–106. *See also* Workplace
Eosinophilia, allergy testing, 82
Epiglottitis, defined, 179
Epinephrine, bronchodilators, 163
Essential asthma, 38
Exercise, 125–131. *See also* Breathing exercise
 actions, 53
 asthma and, 10, 11
 childhood asthma, 186–187
 doctor questions, 139
 exercise-induced asthma, avoidance of, 128–130
 pollution and, 128
 rationale for, 126–127
 recommendations for, 130–131
 safety in, 127–128
Exercise-induced asthma:
 avoidance of, in exercise, 128–130
 described, 35
Extrinsic asthma, 7–8, 17
Eye, allergy symptoms, 64

227

## F

Family. *See* Childhood asthma
Family counseling, childhood asthma, 194
Fatigue, asthma attack, 28
Firshein, Richard N., 44
Flow rate tests, described, 31–32
Food additives:
   asthma and, 47
   food allergy awareness, 77–78
Food allergies. *See also* Allergies; Asthma
   allergy symptoms, 64
   responses to, 69–71
   triggers of, 73–79
Food groups:
   food allergy awareness, 77
   listing of, 205–210
Forced Expiratory Volume (FEV) test, described, 31
Formaldehyde, indoor environmental control, 96, 98
Functional Residual Capacity (FRC) test, described, 32

## G

Gastrointestinal reflux, holistic approach, 122–123
Genetics:
   asthma, 8–9
   atopy and, 61
Grinder's asthma, 38

## H

Heartbeat, breathing exercise, 138
HEPA filter:
   indoor environmental control, 93, 94, 184
   workplace, 106
Herbal medicine, alternative strategies, 142–143
Histamine, allergies and, 66
Hives, allergy symptoms, 64
Hogshead, Nancy, 127
Holistic approach, 109–124
   actions, 52–53
   awareness, 113–117
   diet and nutrition, 118–123
   doctors and, 53–55, 123–124
   journals, 56
   principles of, vii–viii, 50–59
   self understanding and, 111–113
   survey, 56–58
   understanding of disease, 50–51
   understanding of self, 51–52
Hypnosis, alternative strategies, 145–147

## I

IgE level tests, described, 82
Immune system, allergies and, 65–68
Indoor environmental control, 89–99. *See also* Environmental control
Indoor lifestyle, asthma and, 46–47
Indoor molds, indoor environmental control, 92, 93–94
Industrialization:
   air pollution, 106–108
   asthma and, 45–46
Infections, allergies and, 68–69
Inflammation, breathing, 22–24
Inflated chest, asthma attack, 28–29
Inhalers:
   beta-agonists, 159–163
   cromolyn sodium and nedocromil, 171–172
   steroids, 169
   use of, 211–212
Insect repellents, indoor environmental control, 98
Inspiratory flow measurements, described, 32
Intestines:
   allergy symptoms, 64

gastrointestinal reflux, holistic approach, 122–123
Intrinsic asthma, 7–8, 17
Irritants, indoor environmental control, 95–99
Isocyanate asthma, 38

**J**

Journals:
  childhood asthma, 188–189, 193
  doctors office visits, 153
  food allergy awareness, 74–75
  holistic approach, 56, 116–117

**L**

Laryngeal area, allergy symptoms, 64
Leukotriene modifiers, anti-inflammatory drugs, 172
Lewith, G. T., 148
Life threatening asthma attack, 25–26
Liver:
  leukotriene modifiers, 172
  theophylline, 164
Lung damage, asthma, 11
Lung exercises. *See* Breathing exercise
Lungs, allergy symptoms, 64

**M**

Medical profession. *See* Doctors
Medication, 157–175
  allergy shots, 173–174
  allergy triggers, 79–81
  antihistamines, 173
  anti-inflammatory drugs, 167–172
    cromolyn sodium and nedocromil, 171–172
    leukotriene modifiers, 172
    steroids, 167–171
  asthma, 12
  bronchodilators, 159–166
    anticholinergics, 166
    beta-agonists, 159–163, 213–215
    epinephrine, 163
    theophylline, 164–166
  childhood asthma, 190
  doctors and, 152, 158, 174–175
  double-edged approach to, 174
  drug interactions, theophylline, 165–166
  inhaler use, 211–212
  mucokinetic drugs, 172–173
  overview, 158
Meditation, childhood asthma, 193
Mental processes, holistic approach and, 112
Mill fever, 37
Mineral deficiency, holistic approach, 118–121
Miner's asthma, 38
Molds:
  indoor environmental control, 92, 93–94
  outdoor environmental control, 88–89
Mortality rates, asthma, 14
Mucokinetic drugs, medication, 172–173

**N**

Nasal problems, asthma attack, 29
Nasal secretion examination, described, 34
National Bureau of Health Statistics, 42, 43
National Institutes of Health (NIH), 142
National organizations, listed, 216–221
Nebulizer. *See* Inhalers
Nedocromil, anti-inflammatory drugs, 171–172
Nitrogen dioxide, indoor environmental control, 96–97, 98–99
Nocturnal asthma, described, 34–35

229

Nonsteroidal anti-inflammatory drugs (NSAIDs), allergy triggers, 79–80
Nose, allergy symptoms, 63
Nutrition. *See* Diet and nutrition

**O**

Occupational hazards. *See* Workplace
Occupational Safety and Health Administration (OSHA), 105
Office for Alternative Medical Research, 142
Osteopathy, alternative strategies, 144–145
Outdoor environmental control, 86–89. *See also* Environmental control
Owens, Gregory, 48

**P**

Paint, indoor environmental control, 97, 99
Parents. *See* Childhood asthma
Peak Expiratory Flow Rate test, described, 31–32
Peak-flow meter:
 childhood asthma, 189–190
 use of, 153–155
Percent oxygen saturation test, described, 32
Perfumes, indoor environmental control, 98
Pesticides, indoor environmental control, 97, 99
Physical exercise. *See* Breathing exercise; Exercise
Physicians. *See* Doctors
Plant pollens, environmental control, outdoors, 86–88
Pneumonia, defined, 180
Pollens, environmental control, outdoors, 86–88
Pollution. *See* Air pollution

Potter's asthma, 38
Poverty, asthma and, 42–43
Prevalence, of asthma, 41–44, 177
Preventive measures, asthma, 13–14
Provocative tests, described, 32–33
Psychological profile, asthma, 12–13
Psychosomatic illness, asthma 6–7
Pulmonary Function Test (PFT), described, 31

**R**

Rapid breathing, asthma attack, 28
RAST test, described, 82
Residual Volume (RV) test, described, 32
Respiration. *See* Breathing
Respiratory Syvettial Virus, bronchiolitis, 180
Responsibility:
 holistic approach and, 112
 parental, childhood asthma, 178
Restaurants, food allergy awareness, 78–79
Reversibility test, described, 32
Rhinitis, allergy symptoms, 63
Rhinoscopy, described, 34
Risk factors, asthma, 9–10

**S**

Schools, childhood asthma and, 195–196
Seasonal asthma, described, 35
Sedentary lifestyle, asthma and, 46–47
Self understanding:
 allergies, 83
 holistic approach and, 51–52, 111–113
Sherwin, Russell, 107
Shortness of breath, asthma attack, 28
Sinus X ray, described, 33

Sinusitis, allergy symptoms, 63
Skin, allergy symptoms, 64
Skin allergy tests, described, 81–82
Social relations, asthma and, 49
Socioeconomic class:
    asthma and, 42–43
    health and, 107–108
Speech problems, asthma attack, 29
Sputum and nasal secretion examination, described, 34
Steroids, anti-inflammatory drugs, 167–171
Stomach:
    allergy symptoms, 64
    gastrointestinal reflux, holistic approach, 122–123
Stress, asthma, 7
Stripper's asthma, 37
Sulfites, food allergy awareness, 77–78
Support groups, childhood asthma, 193
Sweat test, described, 33

**T**
Tachypnea, asthma attack, 28
Tartrazine, food allergy awareness, 78
Testing. *See also* Diagnosis
    for allergies, 81–82
    for asthma, 31–34
Theophylline, bronchodilators, 164–166, 214
Time out, childhood asthma, 193

Total Lung Capacity (TLC) test, described, 32
True asthma, 38

**U**
U.S. Environmental Protection Agency (EPA), 46
Urbanization, asthma and, 45–46
Urticaria, allergy symptoms, 64

**V**
Van Roorda, Ruurd, 45
Visualization process, alternative strategies, 147
Vitamin deficiency, holistic approach, 118–121
Volatile chemicals, indoor environmental control, 97, 99

**W**
Warm-ups, exercise, 130, 131
Warning signs:
    of asthma, 30
    of childhood asthma, 178–180
Watkins, A. D., 148
Wheezing, asthma attack, 27
Wood smoke, indoor environmental control, 97–98
Workplace, 101–106. *See also* Air pollution
    building-related illness, 104–105
    environmental actions in, 105–106
    problem identification, 102–104
    risk identification, 104

# About the Author

Betty B. Wray, M.D., is past president of the American College of Asthma, Allergy, and Immunology. Listed in *The Best Doctors in America,* she is also Chief, Section of Allergy-Immunology and Vice-Chairman of the Department of Pediatrics at the Medical College of Georgia. Recognized as an international leader in her field, Dr. Wray is a respected researcher and clinician who is also the inventor of the award-winning Medical Compliance Dispenser.

Dr. Wray serves on the editorial boards of *Journal of Asthma* and *Annals of Allergy, Asthma, and Immunology.*